WAKE UP

The Happy Brain

by Great Minds From Around the World

Edited by
Steven E Schmitt

FIRST EDITION

Wake Up Inc
California

CONTENTS

INTRODUCTION

"Happy Brain"

Welcome to *Wake Up: The Happy Brain*, a collection of perspectives from a variety of chiropractors, naturopaths, alternative medicine practitioners, therapists, and product developers, specifically conceived and designed to give you, the reader, as wide a range of unique perspectives from a holistic point of view. If you are reading this book, it is meant to be.

Essentially, this is a practical workbook about how these authors from around the world have in their own unique way awakened to their calling and thought outside of the box to offer positive treatment modalities for a variety of conditions. We believe this book will provide a comprehensive insight into how these pioneers have transformed lives and benefited consumers in ways that go beyond the allopathic treatment model of Western medicine. In fact, I guarantee that there is literally something for everyone, from stories that detail personal recovery and new perspectives on getting back to the basics, to thriving in an increasingly complex world.

Each author, at the end of his or her story, has a personal biography with contact information. We encourage you to take full advantage of this opportunity to reach out to any author of your choice for further information and personal coaching. I would also like to take this opportunity to thank my fellow authors for the excellent work they perform all over the world. It is genuinely awe-inspiring to see the writing of so many dynamic healers gathered in one place to share their unique messages, secrets, and stories. While you read this book, keep in mind that you also have the capacity within yourself to achieve a resilient, happy brain!

Steven E Schmitt,
Laguna Beach, CA, 2019

WAKE UP

The Happy Brain

THE POWER OF SELF HEALING

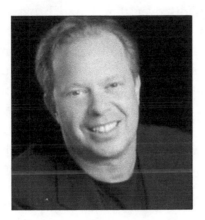

Dr. Joe Dispenza

In order for some of us to wake up, we sometimes need a wake-up call. In 1986, I got the call. On a beautiful Southern California day in April, I had the privilege of being run over by an SUV in a Palm Springs triathlon. That moment changed my life and started me on this whole journey. I was 23 at the time, with a relatively new chiropractic practice in La Jolla, California, and I'd trained hard for this triathlon for months.

I had finished the swimming segment and was in the biking portion of the race when it happened. I was coming up to a tricky turn where I knew we'd be merging with traffic. A police officer, with his back to the oncoming cars, waved me on to turn right and follow the course. Since I was fully exerting myself and focused on the race, I never took my eyes off of him. As I passed two cyclists on that particular corner, a red four-wheel-drive Bronco going about 55 miles an hour slammed into my bike from behind. The next thing I knew, I was catapulted up into the air; then I landed squarely on my backside. Because of the speed of the vehicle and the slow reflexes of the elderly woman driving the Bronco, the SUV kept coming toward me, and I was soon reunited with its bumper. I quickly grabbed the bumper in order to avoid being run over and to stop my body from passing between metal and asphalt. So I was dragged down the road a bit before the driver realized what was happening. When she finally did abruptly stop, I tumbled out of control for about 20 yards.

I would soon discover that I had broken six vertebrae: I had compression fractures in thoracic 8, 9, 10, 11, and 12 and lumbar 1 (ranging from my shoulder blades to my kidneys). The vertebrae in the spine are stacked like individual blocks, and when I hit the ground with that kind of force, they collapsed and compressed from the impact. The eighth thoracic vertebra, the top segment that I broke, was more than 60 percent collapsed, and the circular arch that contained and protected the spinal cord was broken and pushed together in a pretzel-like shape. When a vertebra compresses and fractures, the bone has to go somewhere. In my case, a large volume of shattered fragments went back toward my spinal cord. It was definitely not a good picture.

As if I were in a bad dream gone rogue, I woke up the next morning with a host of neurological symptoms, including several different types pain; different degrees of numbness, tingling, and some loss of feeling in my legs; and some sobering difficulties in controlling my movements.

So after I had all the blood tests, x-rays, CAT scans, and MRIs at the hospital, the orthopedic surgeon showed me the results and somberly delivered the news: In order to contain the bone fragments that were now on my spinal cord, I needed surgery to implant a Harrington rod. That would mean cutting out the back parts of the vertebrae from two to three segments above and below the fractures and then screwing and clamping two 12-inch stainless-steel rods along both sides of my spinal column. Then they'd scrape some fragments off my hip bone and paste them over the rods. It would be major surgery, but it would mean I'd at least have a chance to walk again. Even so, I knew I'd probably still be somewhat disabled, and I'd have to live with chronic pain for the rest of my life. Needless to say, I didn't like that option.

But if I chose not to have the surgery, paralysis seemed

certain. The best neurologist in the Palm Springs area, who concurred with the first surgeon's opinion, told me that he knew of no other patient in the United States in my condition who had refused it. The impact of the accident had compressed my T-8 vertebra into a wedge shape that would prevent my spine from being able to bear the weight of my body if I were to stand up: My backbone would collapse, pushing those shattered bits of the vertebra deep into my spinal cord, causing instant paralysis from my chest down. That was hardly an attractive option either.

Maybe I was just young and bold at that time in my life, but I decided against the medical model and the expert recommendations. I believe that there's an intelligence, an invisible consciousness, within each of us that's the giver of life. It supports, maintains, protects, and heals us every moment. It creates almost 100 trillion specialized cells (starting from only 2), it keeps our hearts beating hundreds of thousands of times per day, and it can organize hundreds of thousands of chemical reactions in a single cell in every second—among many other amazing functions. I reasoned at the time that if this intelligence was real and if it willfully, mindfully, and lovingly had such amazing abilities, maybe I could take my attention off my external world and begin to go within and connect with it—developing a relationship with it.

But while I intellectually understood that the body often has the capacity to heal itself, now I had to apply every bit of philosophy that I knew in order to take that knowledge to the next level and beyond, to create a true experience with healing. And since I wasn't going anywhere or I wasn't doing anything except lying face down, I decided on two things. First, every day I would put all of my conscious attention on this intelligence within me and give it a plan, a template, a vision, with very specific orders, and then I would surrender my healing to this greater mind that has unlimited power, allowing it to do the healing for me. And second, I wouldn't let any thought slip by my awareness that I didn't want to experience.

At nine and a half weeks after the accident, I got up and walked back into my life—without having any body cast or any surgeries. I had reached full recovery. I started seeing patients again at ten weeks and was back to training and lifting weights again, while continuing my rehabilitation, at twelve weeks. I discovered that I was the placebo. And now, almost 30 years after the accident, I can honestly say that I've hardly ever had back pain since.

About the Author

Dr. Joe Dispenza, PhD.

Dr Dispenza is an international lecturer, researcher, corporate consultant, author, and educator who has been invited to speak in more than 33 countries on six continents. As a lecturer and educator, he is driven by the conviction that each of us has the potential for greatness and unlimited abilities. In his easy-to-understand, encouraging, and compassionate style, he has educated thousands of people, detailing how they can rewire their brains and recondition their bodies to make lasting changes.

In addition to offering a variety of online courses and teleclasses, he has personally taught three-day Progressive Workshops, five-day Advanced Workshops, and seven-day Week Long Advanced Retreats in the U.S. and abroad. Starting in 2018, his workshops became week-long offerings, and the content of the progressive workshops became available online. (To learn more, please visit the events section at: www.drjoedispenza.com.)

Dr. Joe is also a faculty member at Quantum University in Honolulu, Hawaii; the Omega Institute for Holistic Studies in Rhinebeck, New York; and Kripalu Center for Yoga and Health in Stockbridge, Massachusetts. He's also an invited chair of the research committee at Life University in Atlanta, Georgia.

As a researcher, Dr. Joe's passion can be found at the intersection of the latest findings from the fields of neuroscience, epigenetics, and quantum physics to explore the science behind spontaneous remissions. He uses that knowledge to help people heal themselves of illnesses, chronic conditions, and even terminal diseases so they can enjoy a more fulfilled and happy life, as well as evolve their consciousness. At his advanced workshops around the world, he has partnered with other scientists to perform extensive research on the effects of meditation, including epigenetic testing, brain mapping with electroencephalograms (EEGs), and individual energy field testing with a gas discharge visualization (GDV) machine. His research also includes measuring both heart coherence with HeartMath monitors and the energy present in the workshop environment before, during, and after events with a GDV Sputnik sensor.

As a corporate consultant, Dr. Joe gives on-site lectures and workshops for businesses and corporations interested in using neuroscientific principles to boost employees' creativity, innovation, productivity, and more. His corporate program also includes private coaching for upper management. Dr. Joe has personally trained and certified a group of more than 70 corporate trainers who teach his model of transformation to companies around the world. He also recently began certifying independent coaches to use his model of change with their own clients.

FOUR WAYS TO CHANGE YOUR THOUGHTS TO LIVE A HAPPY HEALTHY PROSPEROUS LIFE

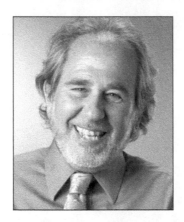

Dr. Bruce H Lipton, PhD

Editors Note: I wanted to include a taste of Dr. Bruce Lipton's work. He is one of the smartest and happiness man that I have ever met. There is a list of his books and website for you to dive deeper into his incredible work.

Globally we are at this moment of diagnosis on the planet. We are standing in front of the doctor and they are telling us we are entering the sixth mass extinction. The shock of this has the potential to have humanity dig deeper than imagined and write a completely new program, unleashing a rapid healing response across the globe.

How do we change our programs into our wishes and desires?

1. Hypnosis

This is the way we learned our programs in the first 7 years of life. During this time the mind is operating in a low vibrational frequency like hypnosis. The theta state is very receptive and we do this two times every day before falling asleep and just before waking up.

2. Repetition

Through repetition and the creation of "habits," the primary way we acquire subconscious programs after age 7. This can't just be sticky notes on the mirror. This must be felt and experienced. This can be difficult if we are experiencing great contrast to the thing we want. Remember habits are by repeating something over and over and over again. Practicing, repeating, practicing!

3. Energy Psychology (aka super learning)

New belief modification programs that engage the brain's super-learning processes, allowing programs to be changed within minutes. Resources to read: www.brucelipton.com/other-resources, and at the bottom.

4. High Impact Events

An individual may rapidly rewrite programs after an overwhelming or psychologically-traumatizing life experience (e.g., being diagnozed with a terminal illness). Read more here: www.brucelipton.com/blog/there-hope-or-relief-ever-heard-spontaneous-remission

What's the catch and last piece of the puzzle?! *Being Fully Present.*

Through the above four processes, we can rewrite destructive programs that occupy our subconscious field. All of us, yes *including you*, can safely and easily rewrite limiting subconscious programs using one of four fundamental ways to install new subconscious behaviors.

About the Author

Dr. Bruce H Lipton, PhD.

Dr. Lipton is an internationally recognized leader in bridging science and spirit. Stem cell biologist, bestselling author of The Biology of Belief and recipient of the 2009 Goi Peace Award, he has been a guest speaker on hundreds of TV and radio shows, as well as keynote presenter for national and international conferences.

Dr. Lipton began his scientific career as a cell biologist. He received his Ph.D. Degree from the University of Virginia at Charlottesville before joining the Department of Anatomy at the University of Wisconsin's School of Medicine in 1973. Dr. Lipton's research on muscular dystrophy, studies employing cloned human stem cells, focused upon the molecular mechanisms controlling cell behavior. An experimental tissue transplantation technique developed by Dr. Lipton and colleague Dr. Ed Schultz and published in the journal Science was subsequently employed as a novel form of human genetic engineering.

In 1982, Dr. Lipton began examining the principles of quantum physics and how they might be integrated into his understanding of the cell's information processing systems. He produced breakthrough studies on the cell membrane, which revealed that this outer layer of the cell was an organic homologue of a computer chip, the cell's equivalent of a brain. His research at Stanford University's School of Medicine, between 1987 and 1992, revealed that the environment, operating though the membrane, controlled the behavior and physiology of the cell, turning genes on and off. His discoveries, which ran counter to the established scientific view that life is controlled by the genes, presaged one of today's most important fields of study, the science of *epigenetics*. Two major scientific publications derived from these studies defined the molecular pathways connecting the mind and body. Many subsequent papers by other researchers have since validated his concepts and ideas.

Dr. Lipton's novel scientific approach transformed his personal life as well. His deepened understanding of cell biology highlighted the mechanisms by which the mind controls bodily functions, and implied the existence of an immortal spirit. He applied this science to his personal biology, and discovered that his physical well-being improved, and the quality and character of his daily life was greatly enhanced.

Dr. Lipton has taken his award-winning medical school lectures to the public and is currently a sought after keynote speaker and workshop presenter. He lectures to conventional and complementary medical professionals and lay audiences about leading-edge science and how it dovetails with mind-body medicine and spiritual principles. He has been heartened by anecdotal reports from hundreds of former audience members who have improved their spiritual, physical and mental well being by applying the principles he discusses in his lectures. He is regarded as one of the leading voices of the new biology. Visit: www.brucelipton.com

RETRAINING YOUR MIND
TO HEAL YOUR BODY
Neuroscience Expert Shares Insights on the Hottest Trend in Health and Wellness – Biohacking and Brainwave Training

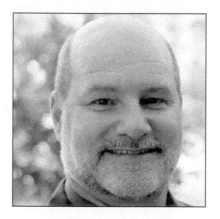

Dr. Patrick K Porter

If you haven't heard of "biohacking" yet, it's likely you will in the very near future.

A combination of science, biology, and self-experimentation to optimize health, well being and focus, the DIY approach to wellness refers to a diverse range of activities including meditation, yoga, cleansing diets, and more. On a deeper level, biohacking brings the concept of mindfulness to the next level—and its recent development has been swift.

Traditionally considered new-age and radical, as it was unregulated, the practices of biohacking and brainwave training are soaring in popularity today, especially as additional research and funds are being funneled into the industry. In fact, biohacking has made tremendous advances in treating conditions like mental health and addiction.

So why do we need to take such good care of our brains? It's just not possible to have a truly healthy body without a freely functioning nervous system (and because about 70 percent of the nervous system is in the brain, it makes sense that healing the body starts with the brain). One way to revitalize and reboot your mind is via brainwave entrainment. Also known as "braintapping," this strategy helps individuals that experience high stress, trouble sleeping, low energy, or other lifestyle challenges, to mentally shift gears, recharge, and relax.

Backed by neuroscience and research, training your brainwaves actually helps guide your brain from an awake, reactionary mind into an intuitive, creative state, and then to a place where super-learning and healing can occur, with the result being a heightened state of awareness and a sharp focus. The practice creates a symphony of brainwave activity and a feeling of calm focus ideal for learning, productivity, healing, and clarity.

Incorporating Brainwave Training into Your Daily Life

Biohacking and brainwave entrainment can help you destress while also achieving physical, mental, and emotional balance. Unlike traditional meditation programs, the method's neuro-algorithms gently and naturally guide the brain through a wide range of brainwave patterns. *The best part is you can actually trigger neurotransmitter production through brainwave entrainment—and I strongly believe it's a game-changer for the world of mental and physical health.*

The results of these methods are extraordinary, providing a complete spectrum of brainwave activity. The restful, rejuvenating effects of even a mere 10 to 15 minutes of the process can help you balance your nervous system and protect against common stressors of everyday life.

So how does it work?

The science behind training your brainwaves relies on four key elements that enable the technology to induce brainwave entrainment. The four areas include:

1. **Binaural beats:** When two different tones, separated in frequency by only a few Hertz are introduced—one in each ear—the brain perceives a third, unique tone. Binaural beats work by creating this phantom frequency, which the brain then mimics. The process of braintapping has shown to produce a state of calm and concentration in the brain, yielding the full effect of the guided visualization and resulting in extraordinary levels of performance that would otherwise take years of practice to achieve.

2. **Guided visualization:** In general, the visual imagery process involves setting aside a period for relaxation, during which you contemplate mental images depicting a desired result or goal. Visualization has been studied for decades and is known to have the power to affect mental states, improve physical performance, and even heal the body. When combined with the other elements of braintapping, these effects are increased and optimized.

3. **10-cycle holographic music:** Another aid to the guided meditation is 10-cycle holographic music, a sonic technology that produces a 360-degree sound environment. In this sonic environment, visualizations become more real to the mind, helping you take full advantage of the power of visualization by creating a more receptive learning state.

4. **Isochronic tones:** Isochronic tones are equal intensity pulses of sound separated by an interval of silence. They turn on and off rapidly, but the speed depends on the desired brain frequency. The discrete nature of isochronic tones makes them particularly easy for the brain to follow.

Never Underestimate the Power of Your Mind

The bottom line is that biohacking and brainwave training are all about open access to science and what works for each individual's unique needs. And when it comes to our health, we are each our own best advocate.

One crucial point to keep in mind with regards to brain entrainment is that in many cases, it takes more than a one-and-done strategy to heal and retrain brainwaves. Yet, with regular daily brain entrainment practice, you can create a path that will help you travel on life's journey in a more connected and more fulfilling way.

Balance Brainwaves with Technology

The BrainTap Pro app uses brainwave entrainment, which is a powerful method of using sounds to alter your brain state. You see, our brains operate at different wavelengths and higher frequencies are in tune with higher levels of alertness, and vice-versa.

Science has been able to link the four brainwave states to improving memory, learning, energy levels, and more. Since we can't sense our own brainwaves, it's extremely difficult to control them. This is where brainwave entrainment comes into play.

Our brains follow cues from outside stimuli, and brainwaves mimic the pulse rates of the sounds we expose it to. So, by creating tracks that pulse sound waves at a desired frequency, we can effectively guide our brain into that state. In layman's terms, by listening to the BrainTap Pro app with its unique brainwave frequency audio sessions, we can literally slip our brain into a state of feeling calm, alert, focused, energized, and the list goes on. Pretty cool, right!?

Neurohormonal Change

When using the BrainTap Pro app, a number of neurotransmitters are being produced. These neurotransmitters are responsible for:

- **Reduced stress and anxiety**
- **Better sleep habits**
- **Increased energy and focus**

But what are the chemicals that are the driving force behind these improvements?

- **Serotonin**
- **Beta-endorphins**
- **Norepinephrine**

People with depressed mood have low levels of serotonin and norepinephrine. Stimulation from the BrainTap Pro app boosts brain levels of serotonin, beta-endorphins, and norepinephrine to improve overall well-being.

Maintaining Brain Plasticity

Research shows that as we use our brains, they grow and change, thanks to neuroplasticity—the brain's ability to adapt and change when we learn new information.

When using the BrainTap Pro app, you learn new things and will begin to think in new ways, making your brain fire in different sequences, patterns, and combinations. That is, you are activating many diverse networks of neurons in different ways. Whenever you make your brain work differently, you're changing your mind. As you begin to think outside the box, new thoughts should lead to new choices, new behaviors, new experiences, and new emotions. In turn, this will also change your identity.

The BrainTap Pro app can help you break free from the chains of hardwired programming and conditioning that keeps you the same. The sessions help impart new knowledge, because when you learn vital information about yourself or your life, you have more raw materials to make the brain work in new and different ways. You begin to think about and perceive reality differently, because you begin to see your life through the lens of a new mind.

Cerebral Blood Flow

Using the BrainTap Pro app helps increase cerebral blood flow (CBF), which is associated with many forms of mental disorders including anxiety, depression, attentional problems, behavior disorders, and impaired cognitive function. CBF tends to lower as we age, often causing cognitive decline. People experiencing depressed mood usually have lower levels of CBF in the left frontal and prefrontal lobes. Most people use one hemisphere more than the other, creating an imbalance. The BrainTap Pro app works to balance both hemispheres of the brain, allowing them to work in harmony. Scientists call this "whole brain synchronization" and when achieved, your brain experiences extremely beneficial changes in hemispheric blood flow and chemistry.

Balance Autonomic Nervous Center

The autonomic nervous system is a control system that acts largely unconsciously and regulates bodily functions. It is the sympathetic nervous system that is affected the most by anxiety, tension, fatigue, and depression, and the BrainTap Pro app can dramatically reduce the many negative effects brought about by these emotions. The BrainTap Pro app activates the "good" nervous system by activating the parasympathetic nervous system, the sessions will healthfully slow down heart rate, breathing rate, blood pressure, sweating, and soothing all other sympathetic nervous system fight or flight functions.

The BrainTap Pro app teaches us just how important it is to regularly activate the body's natural "relaxation response," training our minds through brainwave entrainment so that stress responses simply can't take over, perpetually maintaining our mental/emotional health and general well-being.

About BrainTap Technologies

BrainTap Technologies is on the leading edge of mindfulness technology with its apps and accessories teaching people to lead stress-free lives. With over 30 years of expertise in this field, Dr. Patrick K. Porter, Ph.D. saw a need for a new approach to help people cope with today's stressful world. BrainTap has offices in San Francisco, North Carolina, New Orleans, and Phoenix. For more information, visit https://braintap.pro/

About the Author

Dr. Patrick K Porter, PhD.

Dr. Porter is an award-winning author, entrepreneur, and speaker. He is best known as the founding pioneer of "brain wave entrainment," which uses frequency-following technology and guided visualization to improve mental performance and quality of life.

Since winning *Product of the Year* in 1989, Porter has continued to research and make improvements to "brain wave entrainment" giving the end-user the best product science has to offer. Porter's latest breakthrough discovery is that the brain responds best when multiple brain waves are stimulated in a predetermined pattern. Described as "a symphony of brainwaves," it is the basis for the new BrainTap Pro mobile app and hardware headset, which are uniquely powerful brain training tools to unleash potential. You can receive his most popular book, *Thrive in Overdrive: How to Manage Your Overloaded Lifestyle*, by going to www.BrainTap.Pro .

BrainTap Tech has produced over 800 custom sessions and has sold more than 3 million books and recordings worldwide. With stress-related health and lifestyle issues at an all-time high, *BrainTap*, has emerged as a leader in digital health and wellness.

Contact Information:

Facebook: www.facebook.com/patrickporterphd/
Twitter: www.twitter.com/patrickporter

FROM TRIKE TO BIKE WITHOUT TRAINING WHEELS: A JOURNEY OF RESILIENCE

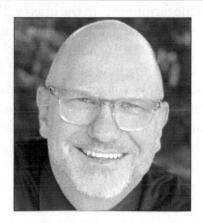

Dr. Russell John Kort

When I was asked to participate in this book, it was just after receiving the award for Innovator of the Year 2019 at the BrainTap International Summit. I was honored and excited and began to contemplate what actually creates a happy brain? As I contemplated this, I thought of one of my earliest memories that took place on July 8, 1968.

It was a hot, muggy day in Strongsville, Ohio. My brother had been given a new bicycle for his eighth birthday. I was also given a new bicycle; however, my third birthday was still a month away. I remember my brother's green Huffy bike with the banana seat, the five-speed shifter on the top tube, and the big sissy handlebars. It was so cool. In fact, it was almost as cool as my new purple bike. This was no ordinary three-year-old bike; this was the smallest of the big boy bikes.

It was a great day—until my dad began to put training wheels on my brand-new bike. You see, my brother's new bike didn't have training wheels, and neither would mine.

I remember the meltdown I had that day. I was screaming and pulling on my dad's arms not to put training wheels on my new bike, with snot running out of my nose and huge crocodile tears streaming from my eyes. I begged and pleaded with him. You see, my dad was a diplomatic man. He looked me right in the eye and said, "I will take these training wheels off if you can ride your new bike around the farmhouse, in the grass without falling off." I didn't give that challenge much thought and just screamed, "Take off these training wheels, dad!" and that's exactly what he did.

When I climbed on my new bike, my dad held the seat and handlebars for me, and we started down the driveway. I have to admit I was a bit wobbly at first and then, once I fell into my groove, I was a natural. My dad let go and I was on my own. The wind was in my hair and I was flying! Imagine going from a trike to bike without training wheels, and I was not even three years old. This was freedom! I remember my dad right beside me as I embarked on my journey around that old farmhouse on that hot July day. The grass had just been cut, and my allergies were getting the best of me. It was hard to breath, and a lot harder pedaling in the grass than I had expected. But I soldiered on, peddling the best I could.

I missed the old water pump... went right by it. I crossed over the gravel-walking path and turned the corner around the back of the house. I remember my dad hollering at me, "You've got this, Russ. You got this! Come on boy, keep pedaling!"

I made it past the rose garden and the big weeping willow with the branches on the ground. I rode by the apple tree and missed the big old stump that was once a giant elm. I was on the home stretch. I could see the driveway in the distance and my mom jumping up and down with her arms outstretched, waving at my certain triumphant journey around the house.

Only one more colossal tree to make it past and I had done it. The impossible, the only almost three-year-old to have ever gone from trike to bike without training wheels *in the entire Universe!* As I got closer to my mom, I let go of the right handlebar and started waving at her… and then it happened.

Yup, you guessed it. That big old oak tree moved… it jumped right in front of my bike, and I had to hit it.

I fell over and when I looked up and there he was, my dad. All he said was, "A deal is a deal." He took my bike and began walking toward the driveway. He was going to put those darn training wheels back on. With tears streaming down my cheeks, I ran after him. I grabbed his leg and he limped along as he dragged me in my overalls and white T-shirt across the grass. My little blue tennis shoes with the white rubber toes, digging into the gravel, trying to slow him down. I actually thought if I could delay him just a bit, maybe he would forget about putting those darn training wheels on my new bike.

There was no more negotiating with my dad. A deal was a deal. I remember climbing up on his back and wrapping my arms around his neck. "Dad, NO! Please give me one more chance! Please dad, just one more chance!"

He peeled me off his neck, looked me right in my tear-filled eyes, and said, "A deal is a deal, Russ." I looked that man square in the face, wiped the tears from my eyes because I was done crying about it, and I said in my biggest big boy voice, "I want one more chance. I know I can do it!"

He looked at me for a moment. I was standing with my arms crossed, grass stains on my white T-shirt, and a look of determination he had never seen from this almost three-year-old.

"Okay," he said, "One more chance."

And like a flash, I was off again. Dad helped me balance and get up to speed and then he let go. Determination was an understatement, and nothing was going to stop me this time. I missed all the obstacles down the side and around the back of that old farmhouse. I passed the willow and that old stump. I saw my mom in the distance standing next to the big, old oak tree. She had positioned herself strategically so the tree could not move in front of me again. As I approached that old tree, I veered to the right, giving it plenty of space… and then went right by.

My mom and dad were now chasing me into the driveway, yelling and celebrating my victory ride. It was one of the greatest days of my life. I had done it! I had conquered the yard on my new bike. I share this story because it was one of the earliest examples I have of mind over matter. I have based my life on this, my earliest adventure, and what it stands for.

So many of us get sidetracked by the ever-present obstacles of life. When that tree jumps out in front of you and you hit it and fall down, do you get up, dust off, and get back on the bike? Napoleon Hill said it best:

"Obstacles are what you say when you take your eyes off your goals."

Over the course of my life, I have fallen a lot. I have hit the ground at various speeds. In fact, I have broken my leg twice, ruptured my ACL, dislocated my shoulder, broke my sacrum twice, compressed four vertebrae in my back, and broke my neck. I have skied out of two small avalanches, been hit four times by cars on my bicycle, had three near-drownings, and five car accidents. I have been mauled by a band of wild kangaroos, nearly eaten by a crocodile, and have been peed on by a nasty little koala bear. There have been numerous concussions, three back surgeries, one knee surgery, oral facial surgery, and I have been partially paralyzed twice.

Through all this though I have discovered a couple of very important truths to live by:

1. Gravity ALWAYS works.
2. The ground will never move out of your way.

I share this with you not because I want you to feel sorry for me. Instead, I share this with you because life is about RESILIENCE. Resilience is the thread that weaves the moments of our lives together to form the tapestry of our existence. It is what we choose to do with these moments that will shape our destiny.

April 1, 1984 was one of those destiny-shaping events for me. I was attacked in the dorms by a football player on steroids and transported to the hospital by ambulance. At 18 years old, I was having a conversation with a doctor who explained to me that I would most likely never walk again. My neck had been broken and I was paralyzed from the chest down.

Fortunately for me, he was WRONG! My C3 spinous had been fractured and my spinal cord was swelling from the trauma.

The next morning, my parents were by my side when I woke up. They were holding my hands, but I could not feel them. With tears streaming down our faces, I told them that I was not going to live this way. They agreed and calmly told me, "Russ you are going to be fine. God has a special plan for you." Later that day, I began to move my hands and one week later, I walked out of that hospital. I spent the next eight months in rehab.

This injury got me back on the bike again. This time it was on a solo 6,500-mile bicycle journey around Australia, New Zealand, and Indonesia. While there, I conducted an independent study on wheelchair athletics. I spent a month in a wheelchair playing basketball and tennis with some amazing men and women.

I also helped a couple of mates bring the first cell phones into Australia. It was a great time to be alive! I was a single, 21-year-old American, walking around Australia with a Motorola bag phone. This baby was a beast—a three-pound battery with a handset attached to it. These phones cost over $3,000 and you were charged by the minute to use them. My solution was to act like I was talking on it. That way, I could look super cool and not have to pay for the phone bill.

There was another problem. There were no safety standards established for cell phones at this point. No one really knew what the long-lasting health effects of EMF exposure, and specifically, holding that cell phone to our heads would be.

Fast forward 30 years. In 2017, I was asked to read the manuscript of *Radiation Nation*, written by Dan and Ryan DeBaun. This book changed my life forever. It was in the pages of this book that I realized the symptoms I have been suffering from since 1999 were likely from my exposures to EMF while in Australia.

We are all exposed to Environmental and Technological Toxins (ETT) every day. It just so happens I feel the effects sooner and more severely than most.

WHAT A GIFT!!! I have been given the opportunity to make a difference in the lives of everyone who has a cell phone. Since reading the manuscript, I have dedicated my life to figuring out ways to live within this toxic world. I have news for you: We will not be able to stop this technology train. We are electrical beings, made up of protons, neutrons and electrons—and so is the rest of the animal kingdom.

As we increase the technology around us, we are seeing more DISTRESSED patients (the inability to adapt to their current environment). With this, we are seeing a myriad of symptoms, which include: neurological, behavioral (anxiety, depression, and addiction), skin rashes, chronic fatigue, sleep, heart, eye, ear, and immune issues.

Most physicians treat these symptoms with medications, primarily for anxiety and depression. This approach to medicine has been used for over 100 years, *and I believe it is time for a change!*

I teach that all dis-ease is caused by stress from toxins, trauma and thought, based on the cell danger response hypothesis by Dr. Robert Naviaux. When we are exposed to these cell danger stressors, biological responses occur. One of these responses is the decrease in electronic flow or voltage.

If you want a HAPPY BRAIN, you must look at what is making your BRAIN UNHAPPY in the first place. Paraphrasing Hippocrates, before you heal someone, ask them if they are willing to give up what is making them sick. I have spent the last two years assessing neurological (concussion-like symptoms) from EMF exposure. It is a personal issue for me as I suffer from heart palpitations, tinnitus, headaches, unexplained irritability, and pain when using my technology. I have Electromagnetic Hypersensitivity (EHS), and at times become functionally impaired when exposed to EMF. It is especially noticeable when traveling by car or plane.

In my clinic, we measure many biometrics including, sleep, balance, gait, cognition, concussion, anxiety/depression, eyes, predictive antibodies, and electrical flow/voltage of the brain, body, and heart. We have an integrated brain-body performance platform to develop a personalized treatment plan for our patients.

There is HOPE. My brain is a happy brain, even though I suffer from EHS. My first line of defense is my BrainTap headset, it is mindfulness-made easy. I use this guided meditation headset every morning and night. BrainTap is one of my secret weapons in developing resilient brains! We measure heart rate variance (HRV), which is an assessment of the patient's ability to adapt to their stressful environment. This assessment also gives me the opportunity to modify treatment plans for maximum results—including my own. In the past year and a half I have utilized this assessment tool, and I have consistently sustained a heart rate variability of a 30-year-old!

Our bodies follow a "healing cycle," which consists of a specific sequence of therapies that we have developed with one goal in mind: RESILIENCE, the ability to adapt to the stressors in our current environment.

I have dedicated my life to helping those who have EHS with my *three-spoke* approach:

1. EDUCATION on the stress caused by "Environmental and Technology Toxins."
2. EVIDENCE-BASED CLINIC that provides a predictive diagnostic evaluation to develop personalized treatment plans to mitigate symptoms of EHS.
3. ENVIRONMENTAL ASSESSMENTS that will reduce exposure of EMFs during the day and particularly at night for my patients.

About the Author

Dr. Russel John Kort, D.C.

If you or your loved ones may be suffering from symptoms related to EMF there is HOPE, our proven *three-spoke* approach has changed the lives of our EHS patients. K2 Pinnacle Health & Hyperbarics is a certified Wi-Fi and chemical FREE clinic.

Please visit us at www.K2Pinnaclehealth.com to book an appointment for:

EMF Education
EMF Home and Individual Assessments
Memberships
Consultations
Weekly Intensives
Telemedicine
EMF Physician Trainings
Speaking Engagements

Sincerely,
Dr. Russell John Kort

If you enjoyed reading this story as much as I did writing it, stay tuned for my next book, *The misAdventures of Johnny Danger.*

WAKE UP AND ADAPT TO THE NEUROLOGIC EPIDEMIC

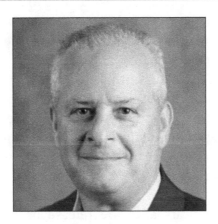

Dr. Bob Hoffman

I have been a Doctor of Chiropractic for over 40 years and I am beyond blessed to have become an opinion leader and innovator within my profession. As an activist, I have observed many changes, refinements, and areas of substantial progress in the chiropractic profession over four decades. I have witnessed firsthand how my profession has adapted to the changing times, to new technology, and new research. Let me put it this way: I am beyond proud to be a chiropractor and a healer doing God's work to help others live their best life.

In 2007, I wrote a bestselling book entitled, *Discover Wellness: How Staying Healthy Can Make You Rich.* A dear friend and colleague, Dr. Jason Deitch, coauthored this 381-page book and we covered America's healthcare crisis in great detail. We offered a step-by-step guide to understanding what is necessary to make healthier choices part of our daily lifestyle.

We documented and shared startling statistics on cardiovascular disease, cancer, diabetes, chronic pain, stress, obesity, and how to adapt our thinking and daily habits to exercise more, improve our nutrition, think healthier thoughts, and improve our posture and body alignment to discover a state of wellness far above just feeling okay. We shared the huge gap that exists between feeling better and functioning better. Symptoms are the last thing that show up in the disease process and the first thing to go away during the healing process. Trying to manage one's health by just measuring how you feel is both ineffective and dangerous. Healthy people always feel great but feeling great is not a good indicator that you are healthy.

As proud as I am for writing this amazing book and for its bestseller status, I have to admit, I never mentioned the *brain* anywhere in the book. Somehow, I left out the essential role of the brain in everything we do and in everything we are, because I had not yet evolved in my understanding regarding the massive impact the brain has and why this amazing organ is so pivotal to health, life, and longevity.

A few short years after the release of *Discover Wellness*, my understanding expanded and once again, I adapted as I realized that as a society, we are now in the early stages of the worst epidemic in human history: The Neurologic Epidemic. Something had to change, and I was determined to spread the word about the enormous role that we as doctors of chiropractic can and should play in alleviating this immense challenge and problem. That was a true wake up call for me.

We have learned more about the brain in the last decade than we have known since the beginning of mankind. We know so much more now than ever due to better technology, more research, and more focus on the brain and the devastating impact of constant, chronic low levels of physical, chemical, and emotional stress. As our knowledge and understanding continues to evolve and expand, it forces us to adapt as well.

A philosophical fundamental to chiropractic tells us that when we adapt to the changes in our internal and external environment, we are in a state of ease. When we fail to properly adapt, we shift to a state of dis-ease, and if we continue to fail to adapt, we become diseased. This truth is as important for our health as it is for our business and relationships. A key neurological core concept reminds us that life is a stress response. We will always have stress but being healthy or becoming sick is determined by our response. Clearly, some people thrive when under stress and others literally die from it.

Walter Cannon was considered the preeminent neuro-physiologist in the 1920s and the author of a groundbreaking book entitled *The Wisdom of the Body*. He coined the term "fight or flight" and was one of the first to study the long-lasting effects of stress on the brain and body, concluding that all disease is a result of chronic sympathetic stress. Our sympathetic nervous system is one part of our autonomic nervous system and brain function, the purpose of which is survival and responding to any stress with the fight or flight mechanism.

Hans Selye was considered the "father of stress research" and also authored another remarkable book entitled, *The Stress of Life* in the 1950s and stated, "Humans suffer from chronic activation of the sympathetic nervous system."

Herbert Benson in the 1970s also contributed to our understanding about the impact of stress on the brain and body when he wrote *The Relaxation Response* in an effort to neutralize chronic sympathetic stress and reengage the parasympathetic nervous system, where all healing occurs.

A.T. Still, the father of osteopathy, said in 1897, "The brain of man was God's drugstore and had in it all liquids, drugs, lubricating oils, opiates, acids and anti-acids; and every quality of drugs that the wisdom of God thought necessary for human happiness and health."

Mabel Palmer, the wife of BJ Palmer, who was the developer of chiropractic, wrote in 1918, "The brain is the seat of all intelligence in the body, the habitat of infinite intelligence which is the director of ill functions in the body from the time of birth to death."

Ralph Stevenson wrote perhaps the most widely read book on chiropractic for chiropractors in 1927 entitled, *The Chiropractic Text Book*, and in it he stated the following: "In the normal complete cycle, the cause is the brain and is innate intelligence. I think we confuse our explanation of what we do with why we do it. We do an adjustment using the nerve rich joints of the spine as our window to restoring balance within the brain where the subluxation began."

If we shift to later in our history, we found the following important quotes to consider and help us wake up:

"The one cause of all disease is the brain and the body's inability to comprehend itself and/or its environment...and the one cure, the only cure, is the body's innate ability to heal."

This quote came from one of my most important mentors and world-famous chiropractors, Dr. Fred Barge in 1980.

The 1981 Nobel Prize recipient, Dr. Roger Sperry, said that the spine is the motor that drives the brain. According to his research, "90% of the stimulation and nutrition to the brain is generated by the movement of the spine." He went on to say that only 10% of our brain's energy goes to thinking, metabolism, immunity, and healing because 90% goes into processing and maintaining the body's relationship to gravity. This is called posture.

The most prolific researcher in the chiropractic profession and the most sought-after speaker in our profession worldwide is Dr. Heidi Haavik, and this is what she said in 2016—"When we adjust a subluxation, we don't just relieve pressure off that particular nerve root—we change the master control system of the body. We change the brain!"

The Council on Chiropractic Guidelines in 2013 defines subluxation as, "a neurological imbalance or distortion in the body associated with adverse physiological responses and/or structural changes, which may become persistent and progressive." The most frequent site for the chiropractic correction of subluxation is via the vertebral column. A subluxation creates neurologic imbalance and integrity and disturbs and impairs the nervous system's ability to properly adapt and respond. Doctors of chiropractic address and correct subluxation with a chiropractic adjustment.

We have to adapt, modify and improve how we communicate the chiropractic story, the significance of the spine, posture, and the nerve system, as well as the degenerative and destructive consequences of subluxation. We have to shift our focus to explaining the constant chronic low levels of physical, chemical and emotional stress everyone experiences every day and the resulting autonomic dysfunction, the spilling of corrosive hormones, and how we go through a cascade of negative events that always lead to damage, degeneration and disease.

Here is the brain-based story that is rapidly becoming the gold standard and the next evolutionary step in the chiropractic profession:

- Stress has been called the "Health Epidemic of the 21st Century" by the World Health Organization.
- According to The National Institutes of Health, 90% of all illness is related to stress.
- We are now entering the early stages of the worst epidemic in human history...The Neurologic Epidemic.
- Stress is defined as a physical, chemical or emotional factor that causes body and brain dysfunction and is a cause in disease causation.
- Chronic, unresolved stress is the cause of all physical and emotional disease and disorders.
- Stress happens to everyone and cannot be eliminated. No one is immune, but the good news is that it can be neutralized.
- Stress causes an imbalance in our sympathetic and parasympathetic function. Our sympathetics (survival nervous system) goes into long-term overdrive, while our parasympathetic (healing nervous system) function is greatly weakened and reduced.
- Our brain and nervous system were not designed to be trapped in sympathetic survival syndrome the majority of the day, each and every day, without resulting in damage, degeneration, and disease.
- When the brain is out of balance, the body will always follow and go out of balance. This confuses most people because it has so many possible names like headache, insomnia, fatigue, eczema, back pain, lowered immunity, digestive disturbances, and brain fog, to name a few.
- The reason chiropractic care has flourished and thrived

for well over 100 years with such a wide breath of conditions is because when you rebalance the brain, the body follows and rebalances once again. This is far less confusing because it has just one name. It is called healing.

- The best, fastest, and most effective way to neutralize the stress response and rebalance the autonomic nervous system is with ongoing proper chiropractic adjustments.
- Chiropractic adjustments normalize and maximize brain function. It is best to measure with heart rate variability (HRV), the gold standard for measuring the autonomic nervous system.
- The spine and posture are the best reflection of how the brain is functioning and the best gateway to altering and improving brain function.
- Our goal is to find ways to reduce the physical, chemical, and emotional stress impact on our patients' sympathetic nervous system and to find ways to stimulate and revitalize the patients' parasympathetic nervous system.
- Ongoing stress requires ongoing care to neutralize that stress before it develops into damage, degeneration, and disease.
- Modern medicine views the body through the chemical model, but real healing works best through the neurological model.
- Chiropractic is a NEURO-musculoskeletal science, art, and philosophy.
- We must ask the question as to what are common stress indicators, and which of these are you experiencing?

- Sleep difficulties/insomnia
- Fatigue and lack of energy
- Anxiety/depression/ overwhelm
- Memory fog and forgetfulness
- High blood pressure
- Low resistance/weakened immunity
- Digestive issues/irritable bowel
- Weight gain/belly fat

- Chronic achiness
- Food cravings/addictions
- Headaches
- Feeling judgmental/negative/picky
- Cold hands or feet
- Hormonal imbalances
- Poor concentration
- Racing mind
- Mood swings
- Accelerated aging

Most people would have never imagined that some of these indicators were stress-induced, and even more important, that proper chiropractic care could resolve them. This is the shift and adaptation in our thinking, in our marketing, in our conversation, and in our professional branding that must take place to reverse the damaging and dangerous trends that have led to The Neurological Epidemic we are experiencing. Yes, it is time for a wake-up call.

Constant, chronic, low levels of stress has been linked to the following conditions: anxiety, depression, digestive problems, memory loss, insomnia, hypertension, heart disease, strokes, cancer, ulcers, rheumatoid arthritis, colds, flu, accelerated aging, allergies, chronic fatigue, infertility, impotence, asthma, hormonal issues, skin conditions, hair loss, muscle spasms, and diabetes, to name just a few conditions.

In addition, ever-growing lists of people are now suffering from Parkinson's, Alzheimer's, autism, insomnia, Lupus, multiple sclerosis, acid reflux, irritable bowel syndrome, chronic fatigue syndrome, fibromyalgia, anxiety, migraines, depression, addictions, and the list goes on.

This is why 40 million Americans suffer from anxiety and another 20 million have been diagnosed as clinically depressed. Last year, there were 60,000 opioid deaths and more than 40,000 suicides. Additionally, the use of antidepressants has tripled in the last 10 years. It is the imbalance between the sympathetic (survival nervous system) and the parasympathetic (healing nervous system) that is the cause of all disease, physically and mentally. When we are in survival mode, our ability to heal, grow, learn, love, and flourish is greatly reduced.

We can re-establish brain balance and neutralize stress in a variety of ways, including deep meditation, rhythmic breathing, proper exercising, being in nature, having positive emotions, belly laughter, deep delta sleep, and proper chiropractic care. Proper chiropractic adjustments neutralize the stress response and stimulate the relaxation response necessary for healing. Effective adjustments normalize and maximize brain function and restores the brain and the body back to a state of balance, harmony, and homeostasis.

Ongoing chiropractic adjustments creates a functional reorganization in the brain and makes the connections between cells more robust. It also interrupts current inappropriate neurological patterns. The adjustment improves: cortical function and balance, risk evaluation, language skills, motivation, thinking, memory and quality of life while reducing our stress level, inflammation, muscle tone, and pain. Chiropractic adjustments reboot, defrag, synchronize, and harmonize brain function. The purpose of chiropractic care is to normalize and maximize brain function. All stress creates brain imbalance and chiropractic care rebalances the brain. The miracles that chiropractic is famous for are the results of the adjustment, which resets, rebalances, and reestablishes normal brain function.

Earlier, I made the statement that the spine and our posture are the best reflection of how the brain is functioning and the best gateway to altering and improving brain function. Posture is a reflection of the stress on your brain and nervous system. Disease is a contracted and tense nervous system and spine, while healing is an expanding and relaxed nervous system and spine.

Posture is so important to our health, vitality, and well-being, yet most are unaware and unconscious of the significant role our posture plays in our life and health. Most never have their posture professionally evaluated, and this is a huge problematic contribution to The Neurologic Epidemic. When your brain is balanced, it will show up in normal posture, and when your brain is out of balance, it always shows up as an out of balance posture with a high shoulder, hip, a tilting of the head, an abnormal curvature of the spine, a slouching of the shoulders, or frequently standing on one leg as examples.

When you get adjusted and remove interference to your brain and nervous system, normalizing and maximizing brain function, you literally wake up your brain and body to become more aware, more conscious, and more in control of itself. I have great respect for medical care, but it is important to note that chiropractic care is very different. It wakes you up instead of anesthetizing and numbing you down.

It is important to realize that the language of the brain is repetition. It is over time, with inappropriate lifestyle decisions, constant, chronic, low levels of stress, and this negative pattern repeated over and over again that makes us sick and out of balance. However, it is the repetition of proper posture, proper chiropractic adjustments, and proper lifestyle habits that can transform us off of the sickness, exhausted disease track and returns us to the wellness track of health and vitality. The brain and the body have the ability to self-correct and self-heal, but first you will have to wake up your brain and express far more of the greatness you have inside of you.

About the Author

Dr. Bob Hoffman

Dr. Hoffman is the President of The Masters Circle Global, a unique practice building and personal growth organization that has revolutionized the traditional model of coaching for doctors of chiropractic and other wellness providers. Throughout his career, he has achieved a wide variety of honors including becoming the 12th President of the International Chiropractors Association, Chairman of the Board of the New York Chiropractic Council, is a bestselling author, sought after coach, international speaker, and the profession's lead coach on how to successfully run a brain-based wellness practice. His reputation precedes him, as he has successfully mentored and guided thousands of doctors and their teams to professional excellence and personal mastery.

Contact Information:
Email: Bob@themasterscircle.net
Telephone: 1-800-451-4514
Website: www.themasterscircle.com

HEALTH AND HAPPINESS –
WELLNESS MEDICINE

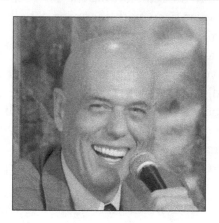

Dr. Paul Drouin

When I look back over my medical journey, I recognize that it has all emerged from within dreams or via meditation.

When I was 22 years old, I experienced a strange yet fabulous dream. There were two parts to this dream: The first part gave me insight into what would happen in my life during the next 30 years. I saw pictures of events about my family, including my eventual opposition to and resistance with the medical world. The second part was a profound archetypal spiritual experience, impossible to describe in words, that I can compare to some testimonials of people after having an after-death experience in which they had encountered and carried on in a tremendous movement of light. It took years for me to put all the puzzle pieces together.

Sometime after this dream, I began to meditate. For many years now, I have taken some time before starting my day to meditate and experience the delight of my own being and its

Source. It is from there that I find the creative impulse for the day to come. Every day is a new creation and an opportunity for awareness and gratitude for the gift of life. No matter what is happening in the drama of the exterior events of my life, when I am at the core my own essence and its Source, I experience an infinite caring Intelligence that guides the whole process toward its greater mission.

Sometimes when I look back on the screen of my life, I am impressed by the synchronicity of events that have guided me. Most of the core concepts I refer to today in quantum integrative medicine were the very subjects I was attracted to and fascinated by early on, even before medical school. This personal journey has been an enlightening process that has allowed me to become more whole and integrated in my life.

My path toward becoming a medical doctor was sparked by a deeply personal and traumatic life experience when I was 16 years old. As a teenager living in rural Québec, Canada in 1966, I watched as my own brother suffered from ongoing headaches. My mother took him from doctor to doctor for a year without obtaining a proper diagnosis of his symptoms. After traveling to Québec City to see several specialists, they all concluded that his condition was psychosomatic.

Once a patient is tagged with a diagnosis, a family doctor will rarely contest or question the findings. However, our family doctor did, and I was impressed by that. To this day, I see him as a hero in that regard. Unsatisfied with the outcome from my brother's visits to the specialists, he took it upon himself to arrange for my brother to travel to Boston, Massachusetts to seek further medical assistance. There, my brother was finally diagnosed with osteosarcoma of the skull—a rare, untreatable form of bone cancer. With no treatment options or hope for recovery, he returned home, and our family watched helplessly as he progressively declined and eventually died.

Without the knowledge, resources, or solution to be able to help my brother during this time, I had a deep feeling of powerlessness. As a witness to this traumatic family event, I began my quest. It was an existential search for answers to the questions of, "Why pain?" and "Why suffering?" Why were his doctors' views so fatalistic, and why could they do nothing to help my brother? It was then that I decided I would go to medical school, determined to investigate and search for answers to these questions, as well as to explore other approaches to cancer and chronic diseases.

In medical school, psychology was one subject that I explored in depth. When Freud left my favor, I discovered the psychology of the soul with Carl Gustav Jung and immersed myself in the study of everything written by and about him. I pursued research in this area during medical school, and it wasn't surprising that he became the subject of my thesis.

Jung's assertion that everything that came to him was from within—an inside-out experience—makes complete sense to me today in light of quantum physics, which describes how objects remain *potentia*, waves of possibility, until they are brought into manifestation through the act of observation. Jung already realized that reality emerges from within. His works on symbolism and archetypes prepared me to better understand the concept of the supramental, later developed by Dr. Amit Goswami, as one body of information in a subtle anatomy.

Synchronicity was another fascinating idea in Jungian psychology. Jung's collaboration with Wolfgang Pauli connected his work with theories of quantum physics. Jung and Pauli were convinced that synchronistic events reveal an underlying unity of mind and matter, and subjective and objective realities. Jung and Pauli sought a unifying theory that would allow interpretation of reality as a psycho-physical whole. Pauli thought that probability mathematics expresses physically what is manifested psychologically as archetypes (deep structured patterns for certain types of universal mental experiences, or patterns of instincts) and synchronistic events (Burns, 2011).

When I went to medical school, I expected to continue feeding this exploration. Instead, I found myself lost in an environment defined by a materialistic and linear approach toward human beings. I didn't realize it at the time, but I went through a dissociative experience where my unconscious world within didn't fit with what I discovered outside through my medical studies. It took me years to align my outer reality with the reality within, which I now express through a new vision for creative integrative medicine (Drouin, 2014).

I had to pursue my inner quest in parallel with my standard studies of medicine by reading and researching what really mattered to me regarding evolution, the psyche, and consciousness. This is what drew me in to the practice of yoga and meditation and to the study of consciousness during my second year of medical school. I had the intuition that these existential questions could not be solved with the mind only. The experience of the fabric of reality had to do with a deeper awareness where all of our being is involved, including the senses, feeling, thinking, and intuition.

At that time, the subject of yoga was not very popular, and meditation was even less so. These practices that many clinicians now suggest to their patients for stress release were described back then as being in conflict with the Christian faith and weren't very popular.

It took me years to integrate these different traditions. It was very enlightening later on when I read *The Tao of Physics* by Capra (1975). Capra correlated the way mystics and longtime contemplatives and meditators described reality with how quantum physics also perceived it. This introduces us to a completely different interpretation of our perception of reality.

Before I could envision a clear path for an integrative medicine practice, I had to experience altered states of consciousness through different meditation practices. I also traveled all over the world to discover that I was not the only one on this journey. This brought me to my sabbatical year in Switzerland, where other medical doctors from different continents came together because of their interest in the studies of meditation, relaxation, consciousness, and quantum physics. As a group of physicians, we explored the connection between mind and body, psychosomatic disease, and different levels of consciousness. We researched and scientifically studied the effects of consistent meditation practices and relaxation techniques on brain waves and brain physiology. Our experiences were later documented in the article "Méditation Transcendantale Revue de la Littérature

Scientifique" in *Le Médecin de Québec* (Blicher, 1980).

Very few people know that Maharishi Mahesh Yogi, founder of transcendental meditation, was also a physicist and pioneer in his work of correlating quantum physics and consciousness. Through this very special year-long experience, I was exposed to his vision and research. This was just before Dr. Deepak Chopra joined him. After that year, I didn't know exactly how this fundamental experience of altered states of awareness and consciousness studies would be implemented in my practice. Holistic medicine wouldn't be known in Canada until a few years later.

As mentioned earlier, many years passed during which my integrative medical practice took on many forms. But there was still a missing link to bridge the gap and bring all of this information together. One day in 2004, I, like many other practitioners in this emerging field of quantum medicine, was surprised by the movie *What the Bleep Do We Know?!* (Arntz, et al., 2004). This was my first introduction to Dr. Amit Goswami and all of the other featured scientists who have since become so popular.

I couldn't take my mind off one of Goswami's statements in the film. He said, "Consciousness is the ground of everything." Gerber, with his book *Vibrational Medicine* (1988), was already pointing in the direction of the emerging points of view regarding quantum physics. But when all of these renowned quantum physicists began connecting this information to the recent research in neurobiology, I think everybody interested in this subject had a thought-provoking moment.

At the time, I made many attempts to have one of these eminent scientists do some work in conjunction with the university I had established, but I was unsuccessful. Then, I just let it go. A few years later, while surfing the Internet, I discovered the book *The Quantum Doctor* (Goswami, 2004) and ordered it immediately. I didn't realize that the author, Dr. Amit Goswami, was the same scientist in the *What the Bleep* movie that had captured my mind. His book, *The Quantum Doctor*, signified for me the beginning of an enlightening journey during which I went through several epiphanies.

I rediscovered through reading this book (and all of Dr. Goswami's other books) the main subjects that had been at the center of my quest for so many years. I finally contacted him, and from there, we began to develop what is today the foundation for the curriculum of quantum integrative medicine that we teach at Quantum University. We believe that within a few years this curriculum will be adopted as the premise for many medical university curriculums.

Following Dr. Goswami, other renowned doctors and leaders in the field joined us: Dr. Joe Dispenza, Dr. Bruce Lipton, Dr. Yury Kronn, Dr. Patrick Porter, Dr. Terry Oleson, Dr. Gaetan Chevalier, Lynn MacTaggart, and speakers Dr. Dean Radin, Nassim Haramein, Dr. Rupert Sheldrake, David Wolfe, Dr. Lissa Rankin, and Dr. Masaru Emoto.

In my perspective, the foundational work of Dr. Goswami has laid the scientific ground for modern medicine and pushed the boundaries of previous pioneers of quantum medicine, such as Dr. Deepak Chopra. The alternative modalities that had belonged to the domains of health spas, relaxation, or personal growth can now be integrated within the medical arena because of his insights into quantum physics and its relation to the art of healing.

Through my own process of spiritual awakening, triggered by the dramatic event of my brother's death, I see today that the realization of my founding of Quantum University is the manifestation of my inner world vision into an outer reality. I had been seeking to express a new and improved foundation for medicine wherein the infinite possibilities of healing can be expressed to allow any individual facing disease and suffering to hope for a full potential of health.

Some of my favorite advice to students when they begin their program to become a Doctor of Natural Medicine or Integrative Medicine, I suggest that they practice a modality of their choice in order to experience the nature of consciousness. In conventional education, emphasis is placed on accumulating rational and linear knowledge through the left brain. It is this ability that medical schools will evaluate when determining which candidates to accept into their programs, ignoring other qualities such as intuition, creativity, and humanity that are so important to gauge the potential of a healing doctor. The process of integrative learning implies that the right and left brains should both be engaged to grasp the complexity of concepts that the mind alone cannot grasp. Consciousness can't be reduced to a linear understanding but needs to be experienced daily as the student accumulates new information.

Having a technique of meditation that allows one to transcend the mind and dwell with the multidimensionality of consciousness will prepare the future doctor to really practice holistic medicine and understand the subtle energetic reality, as well as the physicality of the human being. This neglected aspect of learning was so important to reinforce that I added a Pro-Consciousness Meditation program to the curriculum (Drouin, 2017).

As we learn to integrate the right and left brain, the brain rewires new circuits that allow us to grasp the complexity of human reality, making it possible for us to practice the art of healing with more humanity and creativity. Another important aspect of holistic and wellness medicine is creativity. Dr. Deepak Chopra brought attention to the phenomenon of spontaneous healing in 1990, describing how some individuals, although discounted by mainstream medicine, have experienced a quantum leap, a moment of awakening that brought them to health. More recently, Dr. Goswami explained in a four-step process implying a creative 'aha' moment, the mechanics of accessing infinite resources from the field to heal. More importantly, future healers have access to this critical knowledge that can't be acquired without integrative learning. Universities and other institutes of higher education need to realign themselves with the new evidence from discoveries in quantum physics and neuroscience that pay attention to the learning brain itself, as well as the content.

One of the most important phenomena in my journey of evolution from a linear medical model to a multidimensional model of healing was not only to broaden my toolbox with additional healing modalities, but to radically transform my relationship with the client from one where I was caught in a fatalistic (diagnostic) perspective of addressing only the symptoms, to one of a far greater awareness. Awakening the brains of students to a higher reality and altered states of Consciousness, along with the process of learning, will create a new generation of doctors that can practice truly holistic medicine.

A happy mind is one that has cultivated the ability to transcend itself and experience bliss. From this inner imprint, we can experience serenity and productivity in our daily activities and, as we grow in awareness, observe the result of its creation, far greater than we had ever imagined. A happy mind also experiences daily creativity and be in awe at every instant, radiantly observing the outcome of whatever the Universe brings our way—a resilient and flexible mind that can navigate through life's challenges and settle back to its center.

There is a shift happening in medicine toward the democratization of medicine, where the healing process is becoming re-centered on the client instead of the doctor, which can only happen when the client also wakes up to the power of the transcending technique of meditation (known as pro-consciousness meditation).

Optimal health includes an optimal brain, the ground for experiencing serene happiness, and living in harmony with family, society, and self.

Citations:

Blicher, B., F. Blondeau, C. Choquette, A. Deans, P. Drouin, J. Glaser, and P. Thibaudeau. "Méditation Transcendantale: Revue de la Littérature Scientifique." *Le Médecin du Québec* 15(8):46-66, 1980.

Burns, C.P.E. "Wolfgang Pauli, Carl Jung, and the Acausal Connecting Principle: A Case Study in Transdisciplinarity." metanexus.net. September 1, 2011. Retrieved from www.metanexus.net/essay/wolfgang-pauli-carl-jung-and-acausal-connectingprinciple-case-study-transdisciplinarity

Capra, Fritjof. *The Tao of Physics*. Boulder, CO: Shambhala, 1975.

Drouin, Paul. *Creative Integrative Medicine: A Medical Doctor's Journey toward a New Vision for Healthcare*. Bloomington, IN: Balboa Press, 2014. Reprinted: Bethesda, MD: Stonewall Press, 2018.

Drouin, Paul. *Pro-Consciousness Meditation Course*. International Quantum University for Integrative Medicine (Quantum University), 2017. https://quantumuniversity.

com/courses/pro-consciousness-meditation/

Gerber, Richard. *Vibrational Medicine: New Choices for Healing Ourselves.* Santa Fe, NM: Bear & Company, 1988.

Goswami, Amit. *The Quantum Doctor, A Physicist's Guide to Health and Healing.* Charlottesville, VA: Hampton Roads Publishing Company, Inc, 2004.

What the Bleep Do We Know!? DVD. Directed by William Arntz, Betsy Chasse, and Mark Vicente. Los Angeles: 20th Century Fox, 2004.

About the Author

Dr. Paul Drouin

Dr. Drouin is founder and currently Professor of Integrative Medicine at Quantum University in Hawaii, where all of his energy is dedicated to consolidating his knowledge of medicine, naturopathy, acupuncture, homeopathy, quantum physics, and advanced biofeedback into a model of quantum integrative medicine. A result of these efforts and services was the establishment of the International Quantum University for Integrative Medicine (IQUIM). Dr. Drouin is author of *Creative Integrative Medicine: A Medical Doctor's Journey toward a New Vision for Healthcare,* which details his own journey as a medical doctor toward integrative medicine. In his book, Dr. Drouin leads the way in exploring fundamental questions in Western medicine and offers a solution to the present crisis in health care in aiming to redefine the current healthcare system and remodel the curriculum in medical schools to integrate scientific knowledge about complementary medicine.

Contact Information:
Email: drpauldrouin@gmail.com
Telephone: (619) 861-2124

GROUND THERAPY

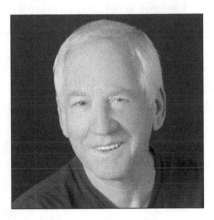

Clint Ober

"The old people came literally to love the soil, and they sat or reclined on the ground with a feeling of being close to a mothering power. It was good for the skin to touch the Earth and the old people liked to remove their moccasins and walk with bare feet on the sacred Earth... The soil was soothing, strengthening, cleansing, and healing."

-Luther Standing Bear

The surface of the Earth has subtle electrical energy. Envision in your mind that this energy is like a thin, translucent sea of tiny electrons that flow freely and cover the entire surface of the planet. Further, envision that every living thing in contact with the surface of the Earth, including trees, flowers, wild animals, outdoor pets, and barefoot humans, are energetically saturated with this energy.

In the electrical and communication worlds, Earth energy is called ground. Any metal object and all living things in contact with the Earth are considered electrically grounded. The reason for grounding electrical systems and communication equipment is to maintain the electrical stability of working systems and to prevent fire and damage to internal electronic components. The Earth's energy is a global sea of free electrons that can absorb static electrical charges or release free electrons to move towards and reduce charges. Lightning is the most familiar visual example of how Earth's surface electrons travel upward to the clouds and discharge atmospheric electrical charges.

For more understanding, consider that every atom on the planet is composed of electrons, protons, and neutrons. If an atom loses an electron, it becomes electrically charged. Once charged, it becomes a reactive radical that can steal an electron from another atom and set off a chain reaction that can produce heat and fire. (This is like the oxidative process of lighting a log on fire with a match.) Once an oxidative chain reaction begins, it will continue until a free electron is available to replace the radical's missing electron. So, in a nutshell, the purpose of grounding is to reduce electrically charged reactive radicals with Earth's free electrons, to prevent reactive radical damage and fire.

Let's now go back to the 1950s when we humans spent most of our time barefoot in the garden, the back yard, at the ballpark or in the woods, running down by the river. Back then, shoes were only for attending school, church, weddings, funerals, and other special occasions. And, when we did wear our shoes, we had to take special care. They were leather. If it rained, we took our shoes off and carried them to prevent them from getting wet, which could distort or destroy the leather.

Things are very much different today; now we, along with our children, wear shoes with waterproof, plastic soles. These new polymer-based shoes were a significant advancement in the early 60s as we could wear them anywhere all day long, rain or shine. We have long forgotten that before plastic soled shoes become popular, we spent most of our time barefoot or wearing sweat-saturated, leather-soled shoes. Before, our bodies were grounded and saturated with Earth's free electrons that prevented our bodies from being electrified by reactive radicals and static electricity. After 1960, with the rapid growth of plastic-soled footwear, we by and large lost our electrical immunity.

With every modern advancement in civilization comes the double-edged sword effect. What is the loss we pay for our newfound gain? We gained affordable shoes for everyone but lost our electrical connection with the Earth. What are the prices we pay for this tradeoff? Are there health implications?

To provide perspective on potential health implications, let us consider that back in the late 50s, over 90% of all visits to a general practitioner were for acute injuries, childbirth, and infectious diseases. Less than 10% were for immune system-related health disorders. Today, with a complete reversal, over 90% of visits to a general practitioner are for an autoimmune or inflammation-related health disorder, with less than 10% for childbirth, acute injury, or infectious disease. This catastrophic shift in health suggests that something in our environment is stressing our immune systems to the point they can no longer maintain health.

Please know that health is the body's most natural state. The same is true for a tree, a plant, the animals, birds, or pets. When unhealth manifests and persists, it is a signal that the immune system is compromised and it can no longer maintain natural health.

For example, indigenous people who do not wear shoes and animals that live outdoors do not experience inflammation-related health disorders like autism, diabetes, lupus, MS, Parkinson's, cancer, or cardiovascular disease. However, for people who wear shoes and domestic animals that live indoors, all experience the above-mentioned inflammation-related health disorders. Further, nearly 50% of shoed people and indoor pets die from cancer, which is rare among indigenous peoples and the animals that live and sleep on the Earth. [1]

Is grounding a factor?

Twenty years ago, many degenerative health disorders like arthritis, lupus, and MS were seen as the body eating away at its tissues. This is how lupus got its name. Lupus means "wolf" in German. A wolf is known to chew off its leg to get free when caught in a trap.

Just 15 years ago, *Time Magazine* produced an issue showing a body in flames on its front cover with a caption reading: "The Fire Within." The article covered recently published studies by Paul Ridker and his associates regarding the discovery of a connection between chronic inflammation and a host of chronic degenerative health disorders.

The *Time* article suggested that Alzheimer's, heart disease, and even colon cancer may be related to the inflammatory healing response of a stubbed toe or a splinter in a finger. Most of the time, inflammation is a lifesaver that enables our bodies to fend off various disease-causing bacteria, viruses, and parasites. The instant any of these potentially deadly microbes slip into the body, inflammation marshals a defensive attack that lays waste to both invader and any tissue it may have infected. Then, just as quickly, the process subsides, and healing begins. When that occurs, the body turns on itself with aftereffects that seem to underlie a wide variety of diseases. In other words, chronic inflammation may be the engine that drives many of the most feared illnesses of middle and old age.

Ridker's work led to thousands of studies on inflammation in hopes to find solutions that could stop chronic inflammation, thereby preventing a host of health disorders with a single treatment or drug.

When the *Time Magazine* article was published, we had been working on grounding research for four years. We knew that grounding reduced pain, but it wasn't until Dr. Stephan Sinatra suggested that if we were reducing pain, we should first be studying inflammation. After that, we began searching for the cause of inflammation. We found nothing in the literature addressing grounding, and we had nothing to go on except that we knew that any pain disappears when the body is grounded.

Early in this phase of research, I came across an article explaining how white blood cells, like neutrophils encapsulate and release reactive oxygen to destroy pathogens. With the word *reactive*, I recognized it as an electrical term, and in a spontaneous moment I concluded the reason grounding reduces pain is that it floods the body with Earth's electrons. The reactive radicals feeding the inflammation are grounded—stopped—like throwing water on a fire. The challenge was to prove it.

First, we need to consider the difference between an immune system-created inflammatory burst (which is health, and residual chronic inflammation (which is not). An inflammatory burst of reactive radicals by white blood cells is normal. Reactive radicals in the body can only last a few nanoseconds before they steal electrons from a nearby molecule to reduce its reactive state. Inflammation, on the other hand, suggests an ongoing fire. So, what is the cause of the fire? Lack of water or lack of redox potential. Redox implies that there are not enough free electrons available in the immediate area to reduce the reactive radicals from the oxidative burst. The question then became *why?*

We coined the term *electron deficiency* and began a series of research studies to help better understand how Earth's free electrons reduce inflammation in the body. To date, we have produced 24 studies, all with IRB approval, peer reviews, and publication. They are all available to read on the Earthing Institute website at www.earthinginstitue.net.

Of all our studies, one stands out that answered the electron deficiency question.

Earthing the Human Body Reduces Blood Viscosity—

Gaetan Chevalier, Ph.D., Stephen T. Sinatra, MD, FACC, FACN, James L. Oschman, Ph.D., and Richard M. Delany, MD, FACC4

Abstract

Objectives: This study examined the effects of 2 hours of grounding on the electrical charge (zeta potential) on red blood cells (RBCs) and the impact on the extent of RBC clumping. Design/interventions: Subjects were grounded with conductive patches on the soles of their feet connected via a ground cord to a stainless-steel rod inserted in the Earth outdoors. Small fingertip pinprick blood samples were placed on microscope slides, and an electric field was applied to them. Electrophoretic mobility of the RBCs was determined by measuring terminal velocities of the cells in video recordings taken through a microscope. Results: Earthing increased zeta potentials in all samples by an average of 2.70 and significantly reduced RBC aggregation.

Conclusions: Grounding improves the surface charge on RBCs and thereby reduces blood viscosity and clumping. Grounding appears to be one of the simplest and yet most profound interventions for helping reduce cardiovascular risk and cardiovascular events.

This study showed that when the body is grounded, red blood cells increase their electron surface charge by a factor of 2.7. That's nearly three times more electrons than when not grounded. A primary benefit of increasing free electrons on the surface of RBCs is that it causes cells to repel each other, naturally thinning blood. Thin blood can get into capillaries and oxygenate tissue, which prevents inflammation.

With the RBCs carrying nearly three times as many electrons on their surface, it allows them to give up electrons to reduce reactive radicles without damage to themselves.

From the beginning of time, our progenitors lived in a grounded state; their bodies continuously charged (-14.3mV) with free electrons screams out that inflammation cannot exist in a grounded body. There is much more to the story, but we will save that for another chapter.

Over the last twenty years, we hear almost daily from people around the world about how grounding has improved their health and their lives. Here is a classic example:

Meet Melanie, who shared her benefits from grounding.

At age 24, Melanie was diagnosed with multiple sclerosis. She had on-and-off bouts of fatigue, numbness and tingling, shock-like waves in her spine, diminished feeling in both arms, and issues with balance. Simple daily tasks, even brushing her teeth or washing her hair, had become challenging. She often braced herself against the wall, fearing she would fall. She developed jumpy eye movements likely caused by inflammation of the optic nerve, a common MS symptom. Over the next 14 years, her condition deteriorated despite medical attention, forcing her to quit her job in sales for a communication company. She had to use a cane, then walking sticks, then a walker, and a scooter.

When she walked, people asked her if she was okay, or if she was drunk. Every day was a challenge, a test of survival. She did not look forward to her tomorrows because her every tomorrow would be worse than her today.

In the fall of 2017, Melanie, who lives near San Diego, heard about grounding through a friend. Although skeptical, she gave it a try. She was feeling awful, physically, and emotionally, when she sat down in a grounded chair. "My mood changed in 45 minutes," she recalls. "The frustration was gone, replaced by calmness. I hadn't felt that way for a very long time. I got out of that chair with a smile on my face. My legs felt tingly. I felt hopeful and alive."

In the two months since that time, Melanie's hopes turned into realities because of grounding day and night using a conductive sleep mat and patches. "Every day or two, I notice some improvement," she says. "I am getting better all the time." Describing her improvements, she says:

- "My balance is much better. I don't need to brace myself or hold on as much to the walls when carrying out daily tasks."
- "I am more stable when I stand and walk. I use the walker less and less."
- "My mood is improved. Much less anxiety."
- "I sleep much deeper."
- "Before I made about four trips to the bathroom at night. After about a week, I was making only one trip."
- "I like to think of energy in terms of coins. I now have many more coins in the energy bank."
- "My' jumpy eyes,' for which there is no medication, is gone completely."

Melanie says that grounding has changed her life. "I no longer worry about trying to survive the day," she says. "I'm excited about living my day and about tomorrow because I know there will be more improvements. I want to shout this from the rooftops: Everybody with MS needs to be grounded." (The Earthing Movie)

"I would like to invite you to place your bare feet on the ground and experience the profound benefits of reconnecting with the natural healing energy of the Earth."
- Clint Ober

[1] "Carol Meteyer is a wildlife pathologist with the National Wildlife Health Center in Madison, Wisconsin. In the past 34 years, the center has examined over 100,000 wild animals. Only 22 had tumors, and cancer killed only a handful of them—a death rate about 5,000 times lower than that of human beings." Gammon, C., 2009. Cancer in wildlife, normally rare, can signal toxic dangers. Environmental Health News, August 27, 2009.

About the Author

Clint Ober

Clinton is CEO of Earth FX Inc., a research and development company located in Palm Springs, California. He first learned of grounding when installing cable TV systems in Billings, Montana in the early 1960s. A decade later, he formed Telecrafter Corporation and built it into the largest provider of cable installation services in the United States. This company specialized in proper grounding of cable installations for safety and TV signal stability. In the 1980s, he turned his attention to the developing computer industry and partnered with McGraw-Hill to distribute live digital news services via cable to PCs. This led to the development of the first cable modem and an increased awareness of need for proper system grounding.

Following a health challenge in 1995, he retired and embarked on a personal journey looking for a higher purpose in life. During his travels, he noticed people wearing plastic and rubber-soled shoes that insulate the body from Earth. He wondered if no longer being naturally grounded could affect us. The question led to an experiment that suggested grounding alone reduced chronic pain and improved sleep. Thereafter, he developed a working hypothesis: Earth grounding the human body normalizes functioning of all body systems. (Corollary: The body utilizes the Earth's electrical potential and free electrons to maintain its internal electrical stability for the normal functioning of all self-regulating and self-healing systems.

Over the past 20 years, he has supported a host of research studies (Earthing Institute) that collectively demonstrate that grounding alone reduces inflammation and promotes normal functioning of all body systems.

Contact Information:
Clinton Ober
Email: Clint.ober@earthfx.net

A REAWAKENING

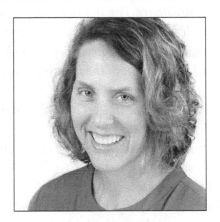

Dr. Alecia Arn

My name is Dr. Alecia Arn and I own the brain-based wellness center, Life Balance Medical Center, in North Central Illinois, an hour north of Chicago. I have been in practice for 19 years and at our clinic we strive to find the CAUSE of an individual's unhappy brain and the subsequent symptoms. Using questionnaires, technology, bloodwork, and listening to the patient's story, we can get a clear picture of the cause. Once the cause is found, we educate and work with the patient's brain to wake it up with chiropractic care, nutrition, exercise, breath work, and technology. This is the success story of one such practice member.

I answered a Facebook advertisement about losing weight. I met with Brian Arn at Life Balance Medical Center. He looked at me and said, "I don't think we need to work on weight loss. We need to get your diabetes under control." And just like that, I was hooked. This man I had just met listened and heard what I was telling him. I wept. He then said I should also be under chiropractic care, so I set up an appointment to meet with Dr. Alecia Arn. We talked and she told me she could help me, and again I wept. That was 14 months ago, and I have healed more in that amount of time than I did in the past 17 years.

My name is Lisa Ruch and I'd like to tell you a story. When I was just 18 months old, my parents were informed I had a virus that had settled in my heart. For the next four years, I was in and out of Children's Memorial Hospital in Chicago, Illinois. I took Digitalis for 11 years. At age 11, I was given a clean bill of health and my mom and I walked out of the hospital singing a hymn. God is good!

I turned 36 in September of 2001. By November, I got sick. I went to the medical doctor and was told I had a sinus infection. She prescribed a round of antibiotics. Ten days later, I was back at her office; nothing was getting better. I would cough, then vomit. I wasn't sleeping. I was miserable.

I ended up seeing her for four months and took round after round of antibiotics until she prescribed a Z-pack with Augmentin. I ended up in Immediate Care with open wounds all over my backside. I had taken so many antibiotics in such a short time that I am now allergic to penicillin. By this point, I had not kept food down for longer than 30 minutes for four months and had not slept, but just dozed instead.

On February 20, 2002, I tried to lie down in bed to sleep. I woke up coughing and vomiting. I remember going into the living room with my husband and just sitting quietly. He said he was going to bed and asked me what I was doing. I said, "I think I'm going to die!"

You must understand I had gone to my general practitioner for four months. The first thing she said every time she walked into the office was, "Let's start from the beginning." I was tired. Tired of not eating or sleeping, tired of coughing, tired of vomiting, and tired of life. I kept praying, "Lord, please help me!" His reply was so quiet, "My child, My time, not yours."

On February 21, 2002, I went to work as usual. I waited until 9:00 a.m. to call my general practitioner. The receptionist told me to come on over. I arrived there and the nurse settled me in the exam room. The door opened. The doctor came in and said, "Good

Morn…" and I, stated with a loud voice, "LISTEN, EITHER FIX ME OR FIND SOMEONE WHO CAN, BECAUSE I CAN'T LIVE LIKE THIS ANYMORE!"

She said, "I think we need to put you in the hospital and run a battery of tests." She said she would call an ambulance to get me and take me to the hospital. I told her not to be ridiculous; I would meet her at the hospital. After all, I had just driven from there. Besides, I wanted to stop by home and get a few things. She told me to have my husband pick up anything I need. I should have known something was up.

I went to the hospital and was admitted. I called my husband and told him what was going on and he was happy we would finally know what was wrong with me. It was a Friday and I had a lot of tests run that first day. First was an echocardiogram, EKG, X-rays, an ultrasound, a CT scan, bloodwork, etc. Dr. Butler, a pulmonologist, came into my room and said he needed to listen to something. He had the stethoscope on my chest for no longer than 10 seconds. It was in that moment I realized Dr. Quart had never once listened to my heart in the four months I had seen her.

Dr. Butler excused himself to check on something, but I did not see him again. That evening I ate a cold roast beef sandwich—the best meal I have ever had—and slept! I was ecstatic! I just knew I was going home today… but that did not happen. A gentleman came to my room and said, "I'm Dr. Pham, the cardiologist on call. You had a virus in your heart, and you need a heart transplant."

My entire life changed at that moment. I just looked at him and asked if this could be treated any other way. He responded by starting to cry, then he turned and walked out of the room.

I spent 10 days in the hospital and was placed on so many drugs that it was impossible to keep all the names straight. I was on a heart transplant list for six months when the surgeon told me my heart had healed enough and was no longer eligible for a transplant.

For the next 16 years, I literally just existed. I really did not heal well and every time I had to have my defibrillator replaced, it felt like I was getting weaker.

I didn't know where to turn. Then I found Life Balance Medical Center.

Dr. Alecia and Brian Arn immediately gave me the tools, the supplements, and the encouragement to start my healing journey. I started with the five-week diabetes program, which began my healing process, chiropractic care, and neuro- and biofeedback. I used the BrainTap® technology, which is light and sound therapy, to train my subconscious brain back to where God intended it to be before I messed it up with this wonderful thing we call life.

Dr. Arn told me I was creating four units of energy a day and using four units to survive, which did not leave any energy for healing. She expressed to me I was surviving, not thriving. The heart rate variability tests showed the brain fog I was experiencing when I first came in; my brain was 99 percent black. I felt as though I could not function and could not focus. To say the least, I was a mess.

I went to the Wellness Center three times a week for four weeks. At the start of my fifth week of care, the Arns offered me a position within the center. Over the past 13 months of working here, my health has improved tenfold. I was an insulin-dependent, Type 2 diabetic and over the course of 13 months of using the HALO, Pulsed Harmonix, the Far-InfraRed Sauna, foot detox baths, chiropractic, and KST energy work, I can positively report I am healthier now than I have been my entire life. Dr. Arn continues to encourage and praise my progress towards optimizing the potential of my body and brain. I AM a work in progress!

I dove headfirst into this chiropractic and functional medicine world and never looked back. I started losing weight. I have reversed my diabetes and no longer take any diabetic medication or insulin. I am down to one dose of cardiac medication a day. I am a healthy, happy, and focused 53-year-old, loving the life I have!

I just want to thank the two people who believed in me and my body's ability to heal itself giving the proper tools, motivation, and love. Thank you, Brian and Alecia!

This story reflects who we strive to be and how we can create a world in which our brains can be awakened to a new happy place when given the right resources and people to encourage the change. We make progress every day in every way. Let us be part of your awakening.

About the Author

Dr. Alecia Arn

Dr. Alecia Arn and Brian Arn
Life Balance Medical Center
13019 N. 2nd Street
Roscoe, IL 61073.
Telephone: (815) 389-7911
Email: drarn@roscoewellness.com

HOW TO PREVENT STRESSES FROM ROBBING YOU OF YOUR HEALTH AND HAPPINESS

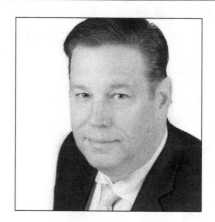

Dr. Bradley Clow

I've got a question for you. On a scale of 1 to 10, how much daily stress do you have? Think of 1 being a beach vacation and 10 being stress you cannot handle anymore. If you're like most people I've asked over the years, you'll likely answer somewhere between 5 and 8. To be clear, that's an unacceptable amount of stress to be subjected to without addressing it. If you're like most people I've talked to, you most likely thought first of your emotional stresses (interpersonal or professional, for example) and may not have thought about the considerable amounts of physical (injuries or repeated amounts of small trauma) and chemical stressors (foods, one's environment, tobacco/alcohol) your body is subjected to. One cannot live healthily with these amounts of unaddressed stressors for any significant length of time.

With your current level of stress, what does your future health look like in five years? Ten? Twenty? If you continue on the path you are currently on, will it lead you to a happy, healthy, and thriving future? Or, if changes aren't made, will it be headed to somewhere far less pleasant, such as further damage, degeneration, or disease? In order to live a healthy and happy life, one has to address the level of stress in their life by lowering what stress they can and having solutions for the many stressors that are inevitable. These solutions must include the stresses you already know about as well as ensuring that you don't have stressors that are lurking to damage you in your future. The first step to finding answers will always be knowing the problem.

I spent the first 25 years of my career focused on helping people with their aches, pains, and physical injuries. I thought I had found the answers to people's health problems until tragedy struck my family. When someone you love, who you believe is healthy and happy, succumbs to what was once considered a rare condition, and you as a physician have nothing in your arsenal to help them, you tend to take a step back. This is particularly true when more and more of your patients, and patients worldwide report a wide variety of other related health issues at a greater frequency than ever before.

It is important at this point that we discuss the term "health" and what it is. Health, as defined by the World Health Organization (WHO), is *"A state of complete physical, mental and social well-being and not merely the absence of disease or infirmity."* Or, if you prefer, Dorland's Medical Dictionary defines it as, "The brain and body functioning 100%, 100% of the time not merely the absence of disease."

Are you functioning at 100%, 100% of the time? How can you tell? Certainly, if you take a fall, have a car accident, or have a sporting injury, you have your physical complaint evaluated. If you're unfortunate enough to experience an emotionally traumatic event in your life, you might seek care to evaluate how that has affected your mental wellbeing. If you are exposed to hazardous chemicals, you go get checked for that. But too often we are not evaluated to determine if we are effectively handling the stressors in our lives, or if the stressors are handling us. Unfortunately, when they handle us, it leads to damage, deterioration, and disease.

When we took a step back and re-evaluated our patients, our processes to assess health and our general ethos of what health is, we found signs of impending problems. The first indicator was our patients often experienced a drop in energy. Our bodies make and expend energy all day, every day. Much like a checkbook, as long as we keep our energy production and energy expenditure balanced, the body will be healthier. However, great challenges arise if your energy made can't keep up with energy spent. If this happens repeatedly or for long enough, that gap gets wider and wider, and harder for the body to catch up to. Eventually, your body will cross a line into what's called energy deficiency, or a "bankruptcy" in your body. The body won't have sufficient energy to perform critical processes, bodily functions become unbalanced, and your brain and nervous system will go into fight or flight mode. Occurring naturally, the sympathetic fight or flight mode can be very helpful in short bursts, but it is extremely stressful to the body for prolonged periods of time. On top of this fight or flight mode being stressful to the body, if it is the dominant neurological state, your body won't have time for its restful, healing parasympathetic phase. This imbalance will only lead to greater damage, deterioration, and a very unhappy brain.

The best way to avoid this downward spiral and avoid tragedies striking you or your loved ones is to get evaluated. Most patients that I initially speak to believe they had a complete physical evaluation because they had a yearly physical and some basic bloodwork. Unfortunately, most physical evaluations and bloodwork panels are fairly limited in scope due to current healthcare trends and insurance guidelines. Today's healthcare system would require a massive shift towards health in a holistic manner to truly become a system about health and caring. Currently, it would be more accurately described as a disease management system. It seeks to superficially address the symptoms of a disease, oftentimes without looking at the root cause. It can offer the diabetic patient ways to manage their sugar levels, but not ways to address the cause, methods to slow it down, or means to reverse its affects. A doctor can tell a patient they have thyroid issues, but instead of repairing the thyroid, our healthcare system offers to either destroy the organ or replace its function with a prescription of thyroid hormone consisting of T4. Often, it's not even verified that the body can process that T4 into the usable form of T3, leaving the patient with no change in condition. Experts believe that 90% of all thyroid patients suffer from an autoimmune condition called Hashimoto's Thyroiditis, yet most patients I've spoken to have never been checked for it during their exams.

By no means is this an attempt to criticize other doctors. The fact remains that the types of tests ordered—and more importantly, not ordered—indicates they are just not looking. I don't want to believe physicians don't know or don't care; it may be a case that the insurance industry and existing protocols restrict or prevent them from spending the time and money to order more detailed tests to determine if each body system is working in harmony and in homeostasis.

So, how does one determine how much stress the body is under? First off, one should have an evaluation of the autonomic nervous system. This can be done with a test that has been around for decades: a heart rate variability test. This test can determine if they are in sympathetic overload, also known as survival syndrome, or have a more balanced autonomic nervous system. You cannot be healthy or stay healthy if you stay in sympathetic overload. This is often accompanied by anxiety, depression, insomnia, fatigue, and many others. Secondly, an evaluation of the musculoskeletal system should be conducted through a detailed orthopedic, neurologic, and chiropractic examination. Thirdly, evaluations should be conducted to determine your exposures to heavy metal and if your body can eliminate toxins through methylation. Fourth would be to determine exposure to and existing damage from neurotoxins such as molds. Think of how many times you may have been exposed to wet environments that may have mold but have never been evaluated afterward. Fifth, a detailed bloodwork should be performed to better determine function of the major organs (including the gut, thyroid, liver, pancreas, kidneys, and parathyroid glands.) As the example alluded to above, there are actually 10 markers that we recommend be evaluated for thyroid concerns.

How do we address neuro-emotional stress with stress

neutralization? The most effective technology we've found allows us to achieve balance of the right and left hemispheres through binaural stimulation of the brain. This increases the levels of norepinephrine, serotonin, and beta endorphins, all of the feel-good, happy chemicals in the brain. These effects are seen within minutes of application by neuro-stimulation through light and sound allowing naturalizing solutions with resulting effects such as pain reduction, increased sleep, decreased brain fog, and overall sympathetic stress reduction.

To successfully achieve any goal in health, we all must have the proper building blocks for the body. In this case, the old adage of "you are what you eat" is literally true. Similar to how one would rather make a house out of steel and concrete rather than plastic and Styrofoam, we should give our bodies the best materials with which to work. Unfortunately, the areas of supplementation and nutrition are exceedingly confusing for most people. Thankfully, our system employs a few very specific and highly effective supplements, backed by science, carefully managing the material needs of your body with how effectively it can utilize them. This means that our patients are given just the right amount of supplementation without overwhelming them or their fatigued systems with hundreds of unnecessary supplements.

In addition to the supplements, we also utilize several forms of advanced technologies to reduce the time the body needs to repair and simultaneously increase the ease with which it can absorb these new building blocks. The added benefit of these treatment protocols is that it is able to achieve treatment goals in a fraction of the time of which other nutritional, supplementation, and even prescription regimens alone are capable.

Taking all the above into consideration, we have created treatment solutions to address and neutralize the effects of stress, restoring energy and homeostasis back to the body and nervous system long enough for the brain to orchestrate healing. To ensure that the brain can communicate through the spine without interference, we use various chiropractic techniques as well as advanced neurologic rehabilitation procedures. When we employ these techniques, we see patients resolving conditions that they and their providers thought would be a lifetime of management to just maintain quality of life. Now our patients are thriving better than ever before by waking up their happy brains.

Knowing how to properly assess and address physical, chemical, and emotional stressors may be more important than one could imagine. Let me share with you one story of many. A young couple had attended one of our lectures and sought out our services. They went through our evaluation processes, we determined the underlying causes of their problems, and they began treatment. This couple was excited to have somebody finally find the root causes of their problems and they were even further delighted to have their symptoms resolved. They were now on a path to optimum health and wellness. We had developed a great personal relationship with them, as we do with most of our patients. During one of the regular treatment days, the husband came to me and asked if I would treat his mother for debilitating headaches that she was having. He related to me that his mom had recently lost her husband of 60 years, his father. This had devastated her to the point that she was no longer eating correctly or caring for the family home and for this reason, he and his wife welcomed her into their home. Shortly after her arrival, his mother indicated that she started hearing ringing in her ears, describing it as hearing crickets outside. Her son assured her that there were no crickets, but over time she complained of the ringing becoming progressively worse and at its worst she compared it to standing in a tunnel with a train going by while blowing the whistle. Eventually, she wasn't able to communicate with people without having them shout. The son was concerned that if the doctor and a patient were yelling back and forth in attempt to communicate, other patients might misconstrue this as an argument. After assuring him that our patients are understanding and caring individuals, we were able to get his mom to the office. She went through the evaluation process to determine the underlying causes of her problems and began treatment immediately and within just two short visits, the headaches had resolved. While this was an excellent result, that's not the most remarkable or important part of this story. A few visits later, I walked into the adjusting room and she greeted me a with a big smile. As I took a breath in to speak loudly to her, she raised a hand to stop me and said, "I can hear you just fine, you don't need to yell anymore." This was a very emotional moment for both of us. After hugs were exchanged and a few tears shed, we continued the treatment and improved her health further. After another few visits, I walked into the room to find her very solemn and with her head down. I was concerned that she may have had a relapse, but instead she asked if she could give me a gift. I was not surprised by this as we have a great relationship with our patients, and it's not unusual for them to bring in goodies they've baked or fruits and veggies from their garden as a sign of affection and appreciation. With a trembling hand, she reached out and handed me a small cardboard box about the size of a deck of cards that she had been holding. I took it, and with some trepidation, I opened it to find it stuffed full of prescription pills of all different colors and sizes. I looked up in confusion and it was then that she told me that those pills were going to be her way out. She wasn't going to live with the pain of her headaches and not being able to communicate with her loved ones. But now, she told me, she didn't need them anymore.

The reason I place this story here is to demonstrate how much physical, chemical, and neuro-emotional stress is tied to your physical health and emotional happiness. It is your future and we want you and your loved ones to be there healthy and happy. You are welcome to contact our office and we will do our best to help you find somebody in your area who may provide this level of comprehensive healthcare. And, if you are one of our neighbors, please call and schedule a time to come in and speak with us to see how we may help find the solutions you need.

About the Author

Dr. Bradley Clow

Dr. Bradley has been a passionate chiropractic physician practicing for the last 35 years in Palm Bay and West Melbourne, Florida. Although he has received Doctor of the Year accolades several times from various organizations, he has remained rooted in helping his community to find solutions to an ever-changing list of physical, chemical, and emotional stressors. He and his team of dedicated staff have spent the majority for the last decade focused on brain-based wellness, speaking to hundreds of audience members every year. He has been happily married for 32 years and enjoys his growing family of three adult children, a daughter-in-law, and a son-in-law.

Contact Information:
145 Palm Bay Road, N.E.
Suite 120
West Melbourne, FL 32904

Telephone: (321) 728-8778
Email: DrBradleyClow@ClowChiropractic.com
Website: www.ClowChiropractic.com

CHANGE YOUR VIBRATION, CHANGE YOUR REALITY

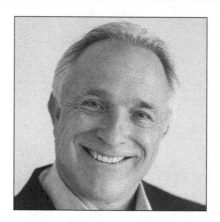

Dr. Branan Dewees

My deep passion and dedication to vibration and sound set its roots in my soul about a year in to my pursuing a professional sales goal for a company I had been representing on the road. I have always loved to travel but that love was put to the test for traveling on my available budget was not easy. There were many trials on this journey, but as you will learn here, they were necessary to lead me to where I am today. I funded that year with credit cards and the generosity of friends who let me crash on their couches or floors, in spare bedrooms, or even stake my tent in their yards when I was passing through. But mostly, it was just me, my Ford Escape Hybrid and the 50,000 miles of road we traveled together that year. I mention the car only because at a time when I would not have been able to afford any repairs, my trusty Escape never needed any—it was a lucky thing for us both! As it were my upkeep consisted of steaming dress clothes at gas stations before meetings and "showering" in nearby lakes and streams with my *Dr. Bronner's*

Soap when there was either no truck-stop nearby or when the price of a shower would break the bank. But the Escape always got her regular oil changes—every 10,000-20,000 miles at least.

The first and most monumental obstacle in my journey occurred a year into my cross-country travels. I had just about reached my professional goal when I learned that the company was shutting its doors with no warning. It was a terrifying and lost feeling to think I had exceeded the limits on both my credit cards and the favors of friends for nothing. And to throw salt on the wound: despite all my pleading, the company informed me they were in no position to fulfill my hard-earned present orders. The owner of the closed company did however give me his blessing to create the vibration lounger on my own, but he would not have the time to help me in any way. Stress overload set in immediately and severely. Sleepless nights and tormented days of both mental and physical pacing followed. Retreating to my best friend's home, I spent three days in a state of self-pity, frustration and anger.

With nothing to do and nowhere to go, I set up my demo unit to lay down. The unit was a vibration lounger with binaural beats playing through headphones. At the end of a 20-minute session, my transformation was astounding! I immediately noted that I felt no stress whatsoever. I was not elated, I was not happy with my circumstance, but I was reset and renewed. Having been blessed to have minimal stress in my life previously, the true ability of the lounger was somewhat lost on me. I thought of it as a novelty item—a great way to nap. But this experience changed that. It occurred to me in that moment that the product I was selling was more than a "cool" novelty item. It was a solution to a massive problem: stress, discord, and disharmony that most of us seem to be constantly marinating in. Now reset to baseline—I was off. I was not going to sink. This was my "swim" moment!

Now able to think clearly and with a deep-seated desire to share my experience with the world, I began networking. I explored a brief partnership with someone I had been discussing the product with. Although we both shared enthusiasm for the lounger, I quickly realized that getting tangled in red tape like a marionette was not for me. The time it was taking to get an idea from conception to fruition, through committee and meetings was not what I wanted.

Back to the drawing board, I reached out to Herb Riehl who had done some contract work for me previously through his company, Sport Waves. He and his entire crew are instrumental in my current success. Herb opened his shop up to me, giving me space, time, tools, manpower and offered me technical as well as emotional support. I now had a headquarters to design freely, explore new foams and electronics and evolve the lounger. Once I had the new prototype, I saddled up my trusty steed! Piling five or more loungers at a time into the Ford Escape, we were off to meetings and trade shows once again with various items falling forward onto me when I would hit the brake! This time was exciting but just as challenging as my first year on the road. They're moments that stick out from those adventures where the Universe presented me with reminders of my purpose and the greater goal.

One of those reminders came after a joint presentation in Park City, Utah. Following the seminar, the doctor I co-presented with, his wife, another attendee, and I went out for a high-end sushi dinner. Now remember, I am showering in lakes and truck stops at this time—so my relief when my co-presenter graciously offered to pick up the bill goes without saying. After the meal, we went our separate ways. The doctor and his wife to their hotel, our mutual acquaintance to her breathtaking mountain home and me driving down to Salt Lake City to find a Walmart parking lot. Upon finding said lot, I moved over to the passenger seat and closed my eyes when a huge gust of wind rocked the car. On its breath, it seemed to laugh saying: "Well, look at you! A 54-year-old professional sleeping in his car!" I opened my eyes and saw a Jeep with trash bags for a top that were blowing in the again laughing wind. The inhabitant was frantically trying to prevent the Jeep from reverting to its convertible nature as snow began to fall. Overcome by a wave of gratitude, I realized I did not have it so bad.

Another time, driving from Utah toward San Diego, a friend called asking if I could make it to Las Vegas that evening. She had friends coming to a gathering whom she wanted to introduce both me and my Lounger to. As it turned out I could, and I did. Many demonstrations were done that night, the lounger was met with great interest and received wonderful reviews. It was a successful detour to say the least. Once the business portion of the evening concluded, I grabbed a glass of champagne, kicked off my shoes, and dangled my legs in the glass walled jacuzzi, which sat some 30 stories high with a view of the street below. My hostess approached from behind me and began rubbing my shoulders. I took in my surroundings and said to her, "Wow! It's 3:00 a.m.; at this time yesterday I was sleeping in a Walmart parking lot and now I am in the Presidential Suite of the Palms Hotel! Isn't life amazing?"

This second year of travel was no more organized than the first. I would meet someone in one city who would recommend an interested person several hundred miles away and who would after meeting them, point me in the direction of a prospect several states away, then off I would go all while hitting health expos from California to Florida. Wherever I was requested to be, I went. I also met with experts who taught me about vibration, sound, foam characteristics, vinyl technologies and many other things to help me better understand and evolve my product. Chasing leads in this manner was demanding, taxing and exhausting. I was running at full speed nonstop.

After an expo in Phoenix, I decided to take a little break at Lake Havasu. The Universe, however, decided it was time for another lesson. When attempting to stand on my paddle board, I got extremely dizzy and off balance. Later that day, I developed a headache and began experiencing intermittent chest pains. It was not debilitating, and I assumed it would pass so I chose to push through it, travelling on to San Diego as planned. Not only did the symptoms not pass, they worsened. I made a call to True North Health Center in Santa Rosa, Ca. where I knew the director as well as other staff members. I went over my symptoms with the center's director, Dr. Goldhammer, who advised me that they pointed to several possible conditions and suggested I come to the center to address the matter. A full workup including bloodwork and ECG revealed no heart issues but did reveal high blood pressure and elevated blood glucose. Aware of my demanding lifestyle, Dr. Goldhammer recommended I begin a water fast to cleanse the body so it could begin healing. Fearing that the demands I had been putting on my body had caused irreparable damage, I agreed without hesitation.

The first 21 days consisted of drinking nothing but water and eating nothing save for ice and the final nine days consisted of slowly reintroducing solid food. I was an inpatient at True North for the entire 30 days and my progress was closely monitored by a team of doctors and interns. Just a few days into the fast, my blood pressure and glucose began to normalize, the headaches waned, chest pains ceased, and dizziness was resolving. Feeling healthier, I decided to take advantage of the quiet time and work. When I arrived at True North, I had set up a makeshift laboratory and health center in my room complete with Pulse Oximetry (SPO2), Heart Rate Variability monitor (HRV), High-Voltage Pulsed Electromagnetic Field Therapy (PEMF), vibration lounger, and a headset for guided meditation with blinking lights for visual stimulation.

I knew that going through a fast of this intensity would elicit a barrage of mental, emotional, and physical changes, and it did— sometimes on the hour! I was determined to work through even the worst of it and use the experience to improve myself and my product. When I had a bout of anxiety, depression, or other mental change, I would record my HRV, then lay down for a 10- or 20-minute session on the lounger. I experimented with various combinations on my vibration lounger, guided meditation, music, PEMF, and light visual stimulation. After the sessions I would remeasure and quantify the physiologic and mental changes through HRV. The results were incredible! I had objective, measurable, scientific proof that correlated with the way I actually felt after a session on the vibration lounger and its accompanying therapies

Upon my discharge from True North, I set out to evolve the lounger in accordance to what my experiments revealed to be the most effective delivery of the modalities. Synchronizing the vibration with the auditory and visual stimulation for a full emersion into the treatment was the major keys. Back at Sport Waves, my HQ, I went to work diligently but with newfound respect for honoring my physical limits. The lounger went through many a metamorphosis in that period. Countless scrapped ideas, a plethora of electronics turned expensive paperweights, and a sea of discarded foam later, the lounger emerged as the product it is today, the ReVibe® chair.

I have collaborated with many people and companies over the

years. Herb Riehl at Sport Waves was one of the first and is to this day one of my most highly valued friends and colleagues. Without his selfless generosity, I am not certain I would be where I am today. Another incredibly interesting design collaboration and a pivotal relationship is between Theta Wellness Group, (my newly branded company), and Magna Wave High Voltage PEMF. With this version of the chair, the PEMF coils are directly embedded with the vibration. This combination provides a person the benefits of cell regeneration, detoxification and reduction of inflammation that are delivered via PEMF while in the full relaxation state that is provided by the vibration and sound combination. Theta Wellness has also collaborated with BrainTap, a light and sound headset. This unit and its application plug directly into the ReVibe chair and deliver synchronized musical or guided meditation with lights over the eyes, which are encoded to the neurological beats in the auditory selections. An added benefit of unifying the visual stimulation with the vibration and auditory is that the visual center of the brain is larger and more active than the other four senses combined. Therefore, by capturing the visual cortex and intertwining it with the other senses, the effect is much grander and more complete.

The ReVibe chair in its current embodiment coupled with the BrainTap provides fully integrated sensory stimulation. The vibrations and sound are delivered through an amplifier that is preset specifically for this lounger. The amp is meticulously programed so as the "full range" and "base" acoustics are felt differently by the body and processed differently by the brain. A voice in a guided imagery has a full range and will feel like a light touch on the skin. This impulse travels up the spinal cord and to the Reticular Activating System (RAS), located in the brain stem, it is diverted to the subconscious where it is stored and can later be called upon in times of stress. The "bass" frequencies are grounding sensations and are designed to get the person out of their busy brain and into the kinesthetic body experience. I call this process within the lounger "Thetacoustics."

One of my favorite things about introducing someone to the ReVibe chair for the first time is the before and after response. It is precious to me to see the change in people when they rise. It brings me back to that "swim" moment at my best friend's home years ago when I first experienced the true magic of the lounger for myself. I recall one woman lying down and having a session and when she arose, she sat up with tears in her eyes. I said, "You must have just visited a place you have been avoiding." She then went on to tell me that her husband who was her best friend had passed three years prior. She had been keeping very busy to avoid the feelings. The woman went on to say, "It's time to delve into it and feel." I was doing a session with another woman who had been going through a tough divorce. Halfway through the session, she removed her headset and said, "This is what it is to feel again." She had been in her head with avoidance, she was hurt and in a "fight or flight" mode for so long that she had lost the connection with her inner being.

I must say, my favorite response was at an expo in Utah. The six-year-old son of fellow exhibitor asked if he could get on the chair. Since I had met his mother earlier, I felt comfortable letting him have a session. He was fast asleep within minutes. His mother walked over and was astounded. She explained that he was an extremely active child who could not fall asleep until very late at night. She immediately asked for an order form. Extremely moved by her desire to help her son, I personally delivered her vibration unit to her home and showed her how to use it.

There is a lot science behind what I have created my passion around; I have mentioned some of it already and I will touch on a small bit of it here. Once a person is in high-stress or a high beta brain state (how many people spend their day), he or she releases adrenaline. If the stress is chronic, cortisol, a sort of long-acting adrenaline is released. Among other things, overproduction of stress hormones blocks one's ability to make good choices in life as high beta or "fight or flight" is about survival. Blood rushes to the extremities and away from the gut while the brain races. Once a person relaxes, and he/she slows down, brain waves change from high beta to alpha waves. This is where we are calm, focused, "in the zone," where we rest and digest. Following alpha, theta waves begin. Theta waves induce a dreamy, hyper-intuitive, creative, and healing state. When we get to alpha and theta, stress hormones leave the brain and are replaced by the healthy, happy hormone serotonin.

Especially for those who create brain stress throughout the day, be it focusing on a computer or driving in traffic, near the end of the day sodium potassium pumps, which are energy producers within the brain, go out of sync. This causes a sort of brain fog confusion and ultimately tiredness in the mind. This sense of lethargy then is felt by the body, even though the person probably does not have a physically taxing profession. In as little as a 10-minute session on the ReVibe chair, one can relax enough to replace the stress hormones in the brain with serotonin, thus resetting the sodium potassium pumps. What this does, quite literally, is wake up the happy brain. When the brain is awake and happy, it then flows energy producing impulses into the body revitalizing it and promoting more overall energy to give to one's self, family, and profession.

When I was 26 years old, I set out to find a profession that I would be happy to wake up each day to perform (I was a house painter at the time). I earned my GED at age 30 while working in the trades as a journeyman painter in Maui's local union. I completed my prerequisites in 1995, and then graduated chiropractic school in 1999, at 39 years old. I loved practicing as a chiropractor and did so for 14 years. I then fell in love with traveling and de-stressing people. I have met so many teachers along the way and feel so incredibly fortunate to wake up excited for the opportunity to serve an over stressed world through my company, Theta Wellness Group. It is said that 95% of all disease in the US is caused by stress. When people say to me, "So all you're doing is relaxing people?" I just smile and say, "Yes."

About the Author

Dr. Branan Dewees, D.C.

Dr. Branan graduated from Life Chiropractic College West in 1999. Upon graduation he immediately moved back to Maui Hawaii where he practiced for six years before moving to Denver, Colorado where he practiced in for another eight years before having a life changing experience on a sound and vibration lounger. With passion and commitment, he has been designing and manufacturing sound and vibration beds and chairs through the company he founded, Kinetic Harmonies, then rebranded in 2019 to Theta Wellness Group, where he serves as CEO.

Along with his own designs he has also collaborated with adjustable bed, PEMF, and light and sound companies to integrate his concepts with their products.

Contact Information:
Website: ThetaWellnessGroup.com
Email: drbranan@ThetaWellnessGroup.com

WHAT YOU DON'T KNOW OR
IGNORE IS LIMITING YOU

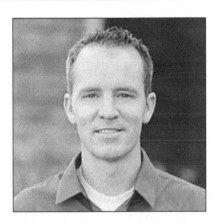

Dr. Brett Brimhall

Several years ago, I was being introduced on a group call and the moderator asked me, "How did a guy like you end up in a place like this?" I am asking myself that question again right now. I was born in a little town in northern Arizona to parents who grew up in another small town only 30 miles away. My dad was raised by a contractor that taught him to work by working him hard. He would tell my dad, "I'm going to work you so hard, all you can think about is school." My mom was the youngest of 10 kids born to a rancher. They were both taught to be honest and work hard. My dad listened to his father and started a premed program with the intent to go into dental school. While in his prerequisite classes, he suffered an injury when he bent over and could not get back up due to severe spasm and weakness. He was carried into a chiropractor's office that didn't seem worried at all and he worked on my dad until he was able to walk out of the office on his own.

Over the next few months, this chiropractor helped my dad understand how an injury he sustained from an accident the year before is what brought on the spams. He told my dad that he needed to become a chiropractor and do for others what was done for him. A short time later, he found himself on his was to Davenport, Iowa to start his chiropractic training. He would study everything he could so he would be ready to help people. Many times, the things he learned was because of someone that was not improving. In 1971, my older brother was born at the University Hospital in Iowa involving the use of forceps and started having seizures. This began my father's journey in studying cranial manipulation.

That injury and subsequent healing placed him on a different path. My parents returned back to Arizona and he started to practice and began helping people like he was helped. As he helped people, others were being referred to him that were more difficult cases and had more challenges. That led him to serving many more people who were not previously treated. The harder the people you help, the harder the people get, and that kept him learning. For us, our disappointments and failures pushed up far beyond our successes.

Over the years, we had to look at people through different eyes to be able to help them. He studied everything he could. If it was legal, moral and ethical, he wanted to examine it. He studied nutrition, genetics, emotional work, acupuncture, massage, hypnosis, soft tissue techniques, light, color and sound therapy, and many other modalities. My dad wanted to know what he needed to so he could help everyone he was able. I was raised in this environment. I remember many times working in my dad's office growing up. Stocking his shelves with supplements, dumping trash, taking notes, studying massage, cranial work, and emotional therapies. He would also have me practice on him.

I later served a church mission from 1993 to 1995 and I realized how much I enjoyed helping others. When I returned home, I went right back to work with him and continued my premed schooling. At the same time, he was formulating nutritional supplements and we taught healthcare providers across the country on the practices he had developed. Through teaching and writing the manual, we came up with the "Brimhall Protocol," the "6 Steps to Wellness."

We have been teaching ever since. I have helped teach and train thousands of healthcare providers and their teams from all over the United States, Canada, and Europe.

I began teaching with my dad in 1995. I worked in his practice doing massage and cranial work and whatever else he asked me to do. I loved doing cranial work and watching people unwind from the life stress they had and how that robbed them of healing. I went on to chiropractic school and fell in love with the study of the human body and brain. I was blessed to work around amazing doctors that challenged me to ask different questions about how things work and what the cause of the problem could be. I remember sitting in a clinical neurology club and the instructor talking about what a headache was caused by. I thought I had a good understanding of that, but he challenged me and invited me to dig deeper. This is where I began to understand and think about the metabolic state of the brain and how "brain fatigue" can manifest so differently in people. Some might have headache or migraines, while others might experience depression or overwhelm. All of it related to brain fatigue.

I did not realize how important that would be for me until years later.

This book is all about how to have a happy brain, and there are many experts that will share with us all the ways to help to create and allow for our brains to be the happiest. When I look at having a happy brain, it brings me back to the Six Steps to Wellness. Achieving a happy brain, body, and spirit means we have to pay attention to all the things that could help or hurt that end goal. Those things are structure or physical problems, electromagnetic pollution, nutritional deficiencies/excesses, allergies, toxins, and emotional stresses. We have created a system to address these challenges to both help treat and prevent the problems from occurring.

The 6 steps to wellness are:

Step 1: Re-establish structural integrity, the foundation of health

Step 2: Rebalance electromagnetics

Step 3: Rebalance nutrition

A. Reset adrenals and the general adaptive syndrome (GAS)
B. Replenish nutrition for organs, glands or systems' weakness
C. Reduce infective organisms in the body
D. Replace enzymes and/or HCL to aid digestion, assimilation, and elimination
E. Restore proper bowel flora to optimize colon function

Step 4: Reprogram the body for any allergy or sensitivity

Step 5: Re-evaluate emotional patterns and remove limiting belief systems

Step 6: Remove heavy metals and other toxins from the body

In order to maximize our potential and especially the potential of our brain, addressing as many of the above as possible will allow us to function at our best. I have seen countless people come back to health by addressing these six steps that many individual treatments did not. The more correct things we do and combine, the deeper the healing, and the more long-lasting it becomes. I want to focus on this concept when it comes to our brains. Synergy is the key. The combination of therapies, perceptions, and nutrients are what allow the brain to be at its absolute best. It is not one thing; it is synergy of the individual parts and the combined whole.

Synergy is seen everywhere: in teams, companies, families, countries, and other places. It's not the sum of the parts when there is synergy in the right way. The results are exponential. The brain's job is to take in information from all over, process it, and then respond back appropriately.

The environment that it has to work in, the quality of the information it receives, and the quality and speed of the information it can send out affect the end process and result. So, we need to pay attention to all the areas of the body and factors that influence how it functions through the Six Steps to Wellness. I want each of us to have our brains be happy so we can create an amazing world for all those we are around. Unfortunately, people feel like they have no control or are not aware of what they can do to have a better functioning brain and body.

I want to paint a picture for you. Your brain has to gather information from all over your body. This happens though our five senses and receptors found in our skin, muscles, joints, organs, glands, and other areas. It gathers that information and decides what to pay attention to, what to watch, what to do, prioritizes the information, and sends the work orders back. This process goes on both consciously and subconsciously. The quality of the information, how it is relayed, how it is processed, and how it is relayed back is critical. These signals are both electrical, chemical, and some are even relayed faster through what is believed to be through acupuncture channels.

Consider if you had to make decisions based on partial, wrong, bad, or slow information. How well could you make a decision and respond back? When this occurs, we get miscommunication, dysfunction, dis-ease (lack of ease) and if that persists long enough, we get disease that can be given a diagnosis. Then we treat that dysfunction or disease through different methods and many times not with the method that addresses the cause of the problem.

Over the years, technology has allowed us to understand more about what happens in the body and we are discovering better ways to influence the body in the right way. The latest movement is called biohacking. This is the practice and study of understanding the complex biology and doing things to enhance and improve our body, mind, and health. My goal and passion are to be able to influence each of the areas I can through natural means to help the body, mind, and spirit to be at ease so we can be the best at what we do, whether we are an elite athlete, corporate executive, lawyer, doctor, mom, or dad.

In this book, I am certain we are going to learn different ways to bio-hack our body and mind, and each one you add will help you get to the next level. The more we combine in the right way, the better. For me, each will fit into the Six Steps to Wellness somewhere.

I want to focus on one that is near and dear to my heart though, which is nutrigenomics. For years we have studied the genes and for a long time were told we could not do anything about our genetic makeup. If grandpa had a condition, we are going to have it, too. But we have learned that this concept is absolutely false in so many ways. Having good or bad genes is only a small part of what you will "have." More important is what environment you put your genes into. According to Bruce Lipton PhD who wrote the book, Biology of Belief, only 5% of what we get is hardwired and about 95% is modified by our environment. Our body is programed to be healthy. But can become unhealthy because of a change in the stimulus or environment by trauma, toxicity, or negative perceptions. D. D. Palmer, the Father of Chiropractic said, "Dys-ease, or lack of ease was because of trauma, toxicity, or autosuggestion or emotions." Anyone with kids want them to be put in the best environment for success. That is exactly what we have to do with our genes and every cell of our body, as well as putting our spirit in a healing place to learn and grow.

If genes were all that we had to worry about, then my mom would still be alive. My mother is the youngest of 10 kids. Her mom passed away at 97 and lived most of her life in her own home. Her dad was 93 and was still out chasing cows in his late 80s. So how does a family with that type of longevity have all the kids die well before their parents? There are only three left and the oldest is 85 and in very poor health. My mom passed away at 61 from a cancer that only smokers get.

So what can we do? What control or influence do we have? Nutrigenomics is the study of how nutrition and nutrients affect genes and gene expression. We have switches in our cells that signal changes to create health, disease, or cell death. The switches are being understood and now we have products, tools, and techniques (and yes, even medications), targeted at activating and or deactivating those genes.

I have seen how important and powerful this is over the last five years with the changes I have seen clinically with clients. I was working with a boy that came to me at three years old that was diagnosed as autistic at the age of two. He was doing 35 hours of OT and other therapies a week and was enrolled in a private preschool. I worked with him for a year doing all six steps. Additionally, he had been undergoing IV therapy and was still struggling with recognizing numbers and saying them. He had a very limited vocabulary and was still in diapers. It was difficult, and I still remember his mom coming in and telling me that, "He is starting to notice he is different. He came to me and said, 'I just want to be smart like my brother.'" This broke my heart. I was doing everything I'd learned and was constantly looking for more ways to help him.

Well, his mom was with a cardiologist who introduced a brain drink called Nrf2 for the brain. She said it was liquid brain food, and the affects were cumulative. She started him on it and a I saw him 11 days into this new regimen. He had the best day he had ever had with me. He sat on the table and I was able to work with him the whole time. In the therapy area, he recalled things we had worked with him months ago. Something had switched; something had turned on. I had not changed anything. The drink was the only thing different. This change was confirmed by both his OT and ABA therapists that worked with him for years. No one said anything to each other beforehand.

Today, this little boy has been using the nutrigenomic technology and he is in a normal school that does not know his original diagnosis. He had been on the principal's list for good grades the last two years. His behavior has improved drastically, and he is now involved in team sports and claims he is smarter than his brother. What was it that unlocked him and his potential? It was activating his inborn pathways through synergistic nutrition.

I have heard countless times that "I have this," or "My child has that," or "It's in my family, so I knew it would happen." Most times, people are not born with a condition unless it is purely genetic, like Down syndrome. What we have in most situations is a system that is under-functioning because of some type of excess toxin, deficiency, lack of activation, or some other block that ties to the Six Steps to Wellness. We call these blocks interferences. Interferences block or limit a person's full potential.

This is a book about having or achieving a happy brain. Here the key concepts:

1. Your body and mind are programed to be healthy.
2. Identifying and correcting the different interferences through the Six Steps to Wellness unlocks our potential.
3. Brain fatigue has to be corrected through tools, techniques, and products.
4. We need to listen to and understand what our body is telling us. We need to treat our body and mind like our best friend.
5. Understand where you are and what you want to accomplish and find guidance.

About the Author

Dr. Bett Brimhall

Dr. Brimhall has been married to his wife Holly for over 22 years and they have four children ranging from 11 to 19. He has been in clinical practice for 19 years and has been training healthcare providers all over the world since 1995. He and his father have pioneered the Six Steps to Wellness. He has been part of teaching, creating nutritional supplements, chiropractic tools, and techniques. His educational background includes nutrition, chiropractic, acupuncture, hypnosis, biofeedback, neurology, massage, neurofeedback, psychology, coaching, dietary management, stress management, and others. His passion of helping people achieve their full potential in health has now been expanded to helping people with their wealth. In 2014, he had a paradigm shift when he saw changes in a patient that he had worked with for over a year with a new, breakthrough technology.

Contact Information:
Website: www.drbrettbrimhall.lifevantage.com
       www.brimhall.com
Office: 480-964-5107
Email: drbrett@brimhall.com

THE MAGIC HAPPENS
IN THE EMOTIONS

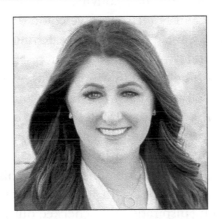

Amber Boyles-Pellock
Board Certified Naturopathic Doctor

Have you ever wanted something so badly but felt it was just out of reach? I mean, you're doing everything you can to make things happen. You're thinking about "it" 24/7; you're making lists, you're praying, and imagining what life will be like once you have "it." Yeah, me too! My story went a little—or exactly—like this.

I had completed school and was ready to hang my shingle. The only problem was I had no business name or logo. You might say, "So what's the problem?" Well, I'm a visual person and needed a snazzy logo to be inspired—and I had nothing. So I did what any Type A, impatient person would do: I asked for help! There must be a way to speed up this process, right?

I made an appointment with my practitioner and left with a 4x4 white Post-it Note with the following affirmation: *"Infinite Spirit open the way for the Divine design of my life to manifest: Let the genius within me now be released, let me see clearly the perfect plan.*" What was released was not the *genius within me*; I can assure you of that! I was on the receiving end of the worst case of food poisoning imaginable! I remember lying on the cold floor of my bathroom in tears. I was supposed to see the plan clearly. How in the world does sitting here praying to the porcelain god fit into my divine design? Something had gone terribly wrong!

Let me back up about eight years. This is the mind-blowing part, so pay attention! I had convinced my husband to extend his conference in San Francisco so we could drive up the Pacific Coast Highway. I wanted to go whale watching in Monterey Bay and spend some time in Big Sur. After a successful whale watching tour and a beautiful evening in Monterey, we were up and ready to hit Pebble Beach on our way to Big Sur, but not before I got my morning coffee. Next to our hotel was this quaint coffee shop. Mike went to get the car, and I went to grab a cup of coffee for the drive. As soon as I walked in, there was a display of coffee mugs. Two caught my attention. One was turquoise and the other lavender; each was printed with a profound statement. (I'm a sucker for anything inspirational.) I checked out with my two new mugs, cup of coffee, and we headed to Big Sur.

The rest of the trip was magical, but that's not the important part. Back to coffee! If you're a coffee drinker, you probably have your absolute favorite mug, meaning that unless the dishwasher is running at the exact time you pour your coffee, you will find a way to drink out of that mug every day. Well, for me that was the turquoise mug. I drank my coffee out of that mug every single morning. It felt good around my hands. The heat of the coffee warmed my hands on cold mornings. It was smooth against my lips. It just felt good. It felt right. I was drawn to this mug day-after-day for years.

All right, now back to recovering from food poisoning. Even if you haven't had food poisoning, if you've ever had the flu or been sick to your stomach, you know what it's like to realize you're hungry but scared to eat. This is where I was days later. I was over the crackers and water and found myself craving a cup of coffee. Let's be real—I was scared! I wasn't sure my stomach could handle the coffee. This was a real decision. After being sick for days, the last thing I wanted was to take a step backwards.

I did it! I hit the brew button, took my favorite mug out of the cabinet, and set it squarely in front of the coffee pot. I was still so weak. I sat at the kitchen island, folded my arms, and rested my head. I was focused on my mug and the sound of the coffee dripping into the carafe. I was just waiting for the beep to let me know my perfect cup of joe was done. In that very quiet moment for the first time—maybe ever—I realized what was printed on my coffee mug. It said, "Live in Wellness." I remember reading that and saying it out loud: "Live in Wellness… Live in Wellness," over and over again. That was it! Live In Wellness; that was my inspiration. That was supposed to be the name of my business. That was my divine design! When I got up from the island and grabbed my mug (which I had done hundreds of times before), I turned it around to read and attempted to comprehend what was printed on the back. It read, "The Universe Knows."

Cue the waterworks because I sat there and cried and cried, and then cried some more. I immediately knew the food poisoning forced me to get all the chatter out of my head so I could see what had been in front of me every single morning for years. My perfect plan had been set in motion the moment I bought the coffee mug from that quaint shop in California years earlier.

Within an hour, I purchased the domain name for my website, created a Facebook page, and contacted my graphic artist to start on my logo. In the aftermath of being so sick, Live in Wellness was created and launched in a matter of weeks. I have been humbled and honored to work with so many clients on their wellness journey ever since. I'm forever grateful for that trip to California, my coffee mug, my practitioner, my affirmation, my inspiration, business name, and yes, my food poisoning!

So, what does your brain need to be happy? Definitely not food poisoning. The brain needs to be emotionally balanced. Many experts believe a healthy brain, and therefore a happy one, can regulate emotions. I work with clients to assist their brain in balancing emotions. This includes balancing the conscious and subconscious areas of the brain. You may be asking, "How would one do that?" We balance the brain by identifying the emotional baggage that needs to be released. I know this sounds crazy, but it's a very real thing.

In my practice, I see a variety of clients. Some want to remain healthy. Some have exhausted all known medical options, and others have played Let's Stump the Medical Doctor and find themselves on my table. The latter scenario is the one that usually has the biggest emotional component. Let's be honest; when was the last time your medical doctor told you that you may have some trapped emotions in your subconscious that are causing you problems? If they have, you've found a diamond in the rough and you should consider yourself very lucky. For you, the reader who is completely lost right now, let me demonstrate what I'm talking about. I always say, "The magic happens in the emotions!"

Anyone have a tissue?

On May 23, 2017, this sweet girl with blond hair and freckles walked into my office. I quickly learned that this day was her ninth birthday. She appeared to be somewhat skeptical and reserved: this child was an old soul in a cute new dress. I recognized this about her immediately, and once she felt comfortable, she had no issue telling me her problem. Her nose ran 24/7. This had been the case as long as she could remember. She traveled with boxes of tissues and there were boxes in all of the family cars. They were placed all over her house, and on the first day of school, she took the Costco-sized pack into her classroom. It had been an issue for so long that her family and friends had come to the conclusion that her nose just runs.

She was no-nonsense and to the point—a girl after my own heart. I finally got around to asking the question I ask everyone on his or her first visit: "If we could fix anything that would improve the quality of your life, what would it be?" She looked at me with those blue eyes in a way that clearly demonstrated she was annoyed with my question. She kept her composure and very articulately stated she would like her nose to stop running. I said, "Let's get to work and see if we can fix this for your birthday!" Her eyes were bright and wide as if to say, *yes, let's do it*. However, her arms were crossed, and her body language suggested that smarter people than I have attempted to solve this problem, and all had failed.

I centered myself while setting the intention to identify and clear any emotion(s) that could be causing this sweet girl's nose to run nonstop. I identified the emotions that were causing her subconscious to work overtime, resulting in a nose that was constantly running.

She had three emotions that were trapped at four years old. Yes, you read that correctly. Four years old! We identified terror, resentment, and peeved. What could have happened to an innocent child at four that resulted in such adultlike emotions, causing a constant runny nose? Well, this girl suddenly and tragically lost her father when she was four years old. Think about this situation and the emotions identified from the perspective of a preschooler. All she knew was that daddy had kissed her good-bye, told her he loved her, and then she learned he was never coming home.

Taken back by what came up, my next challenge was to get her to think about the worst day of her life on her birthday. I remember she attacked this task like a champ! I asked, "Did something bad happen when you were four?" Her head dropped, and her voice quivered, and I will never forget the words she said next. She looked at me, fighting back tears and said, "My daddy died when I was four!" To be honest, we were all fighting back tears. Now I have to push this already emotional child a bit further. We had to break down these three emotions individually in order to release them. Her mom and I sat there as she recounted the terror she felt the day her daddy died. Then without even realizing it, she described the peeved and resentment as she continued to recall that horrific day in her own words. "It wasn't fair! Why did my daddy have to die?"

After clearing these emotions by going to a very dark day, she lifted her head, and with tears in her eyes said, "Are we done now?" She wasn't complaining. This girl merely asked because that's just who she is and how she rolls. I was so thankful to be able to answer with an overwhelming "Yes!"

Within days of clearing these emotions, her nose stopped running. She knew immediately things were better, but I think her mom and the rest of family were waiting for the proverbial other shoe to drop. How could something as simple as clearing a few emotions from the most traumatic day of her life stop a nose from running? It's simple: her subconscious and conscious brain were balanced.

When this girl learned of her father's death, lots of tears were shed. Those tears continued for days, months, and years! The subconscious is always trying to protect us, but sometimes it can be overprotective. This little girl grew up way to quickly by learning life is not guaranteed, and bad things can happen to good people.

We all have past emotions, events, traumas, etc. that have hurt us emotionally. It's if, when, and how we decide to deal with the past hurts and associated emotions that has such a huge impact on our brain. Consciously, this little girl wanted nothing more than for her nose to stop running. Clearly, that wasn't enough. It wasn't until we asked the subconscious for answers that we were able to resolve the issue.

In the words of a nine-year-old, "Did you know my nose ran all the time because daddy died… and now, it doesn't?"

Baby Wanted

One June day, this beautiful girl walked into my office. You know the type: every hair in place, the perfect smoky eye, wearing the cutest outfit ever.

"I've tried for nine months to get pregnant, and nothing has worked, and I'm a very emotional person." I had already learned not to ask questions with obvious answers. So she wanted help getting pregnant. Got it! I started with a balancing treatment and we identified several emotions that were trapped. We found crying, hatred, and self-abuse, and all needed to be released during that visit. We talked about when each one was trapped and circumstances surrounding the emotions, clearing them one by one.

We traced the hatred back to some family drama eight years earlier. She had no qualms admitting she wasn't over this emotional pain and thought about the situation often. After clearing hatred, she asked me if I could find out where that emotion had been trapped. I replied, "Let's ask." That emotion had been trapped in her uterus. This client conceived four days later and now has a happy, healthy, and growing baby boy!

If you want to have a happy brain, you must make sure both parts are balanced! Like I always say, "The *magic* happens in the emotions!"

About the Author

Amber Boyles-Pellock

Amber is a traditional naturopath who is board certified by the American Naturopathic Medical Certification Board and is also board certified in holistic nutrition. She has attended various educational institutions including the Food Enzyme Institute, Trinity School of Natural Health, the University of Western States in Oregon, and the Institute of Transformational Nutrition in Los Angeles. In January 2017, she opened her own practice, Live In Wellness, in Edwardsville, IL.

She thinks of herself as a holistic health detective who keeps digging to find answers in order to help her clients. She uses her education and experience in combination with various modalities to help her clients achieve wellness in all parts of life. Boyles-Pellock is still on her journey to wellness and everyday strives for self-improvement. She feels that it is her calling to help others do the same.

Contact Information:
Live In Wellness
2 Club Centre Court, Suite 3
Edwardsville, IL 62025
618-391-0605
amber@ILiveInWellness.com

INFINITE DANCE

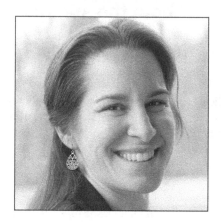

Dr. Carly Sorrell

Since I was little, I've wanted to help people and always knew there was much more to our existence than we can comprehend. I grew up wanting to become a pediatric surgeon. I was fortunate enough to be able to observe some surgeries, just to have the surgeon laugh at me when I told him I wanted to become a doctor to help people. Being an optimist, I didn't let that deter me from pursuing my dream. When I was 12 years old, I experienced back pain and went to a physical therapist for treatment, had some relief, but didn't feel like it was helping. From then my pain would come and go; I wore a support belt from time to time just dealing with it, not knowing something more serious was happening on the inside of my body.

As time went on, I entered the wonderful world of cramps as puberty hit. However, not accepting this was a beautiful time of natural self-transformation, the only thing that went through my mind was, "Why am I a girl? Why do I have to wear a bra and what felt like a diaper in my underwear every month!?" My cramps were incredibly painful like my back pain, only they were in the front, so I either dealt with it or took a pill to cover it up. There were times where I just wanted to lay on the couch in the fetal position. I also started having headaches all the time, and later came the next set of symptoms. With irritable bowel syndrome, I didn't feel stressed but maybe my back pain, cramps, headaches, and things I wanted to say but didn't were piece of what was causing my bowels to tighten right up.

I thought I was happy, but on the inside I was not. Our body is aware and remembers everything happening to it, whether we are consciously in tune to it or not. Symptoms are warning signs that something isn't right, and covering up symptoms is like wearing a mask, not allowing it to fully express itself. It's best to first look at the control center of our body to see if there's an interference somewhere. Our brain and nervous system control and coordinate every cell of our body, meaning our brain is in constant communication with every part of our body, so we can do the things we are meant to do and adapt to our environment the best way possible.

By the age of 16, my cramps continued to become worse. After my first penetrating experience at the gynecologist, I was told I had a tilted uterus and because of my painful cramps, he wanted to take a deeper look with laparoscopy surgery just to find endometriosis. I went on the birth control pill and he told me it's harder to get pregnant when you have endometriosis. This was not an issue at the time, but it struck a chord with me since I've always wanted to have kids. About a year and half later, I had an abnormal pap smear, which lead to having a biopsy of my cervix. I thought this must have been similar to medieval torture as chunks of tissue were being ripped out of me, all while the nurse said, "It shouldn't be hurting," as tears streamed down my face. I'm nearly broke my mom's hand from squeezing it so hard. From there, they freeze-dried my cervix to kill any pre-cancerous cells along with who knows how many good ones.

Thoughts ran through my brain like, "What's wrong with my body?" and, "Why one thing after another?" I came to just expect something else to happen every year or two. Over the years, the thoughts I had were to expect something to go wrong at that interval. This is a perfect example of how our thought control has a tremendous impact on our body. I was already predicting illness and my thoughts were a contributing factor for something to occur down the road. Each cell of our body is in continuous vibration and we can choose to vibrate high or low, in harmony or in chaos with our thoughts, which is the one thing we do have control of, and no one else. My brain was vibrating low, in chaos expecting something to go wrong.

Our Divine Source always offers doors of opportunity; we just need to take the time to stop, listen and trust. During high school, my boyfriend at the time had been to a chiropractor his whole life and kept telling me to go, probably because he was tired of hearing me complain. The reason why I didn't go is because it was unfamiliar, which brought on fear, so I resorted to staying in the same type of treatment with which I was comfortable. Ironically, I continued to get worse not only in my back, but my entire body. I was in survival mode with a symptom-treated body. One day when my back pain returned with a vengeance, it was difficult to even walk. So, finally I went to a chiropractor.

I had no idea how different life would be under chiropractic care! This was my physical body waking up! It was like nothing I ever felt before, as if someone turned the lights on inside me! Just like turning the dimmer switch up, I had no idea I was living life with such a dim light. I thought, "What did this chiropractor do?" What he did was adjust the bones in my spine to relieve the pressure put on the nerves coming off my spine that branch off traveling to every cell of our body. That someone that I felt turning the lights on brighter was me. It was my internal healing ability turning on even more, known as my Innate Intelligence. Our Innate Intelligence is our spark of life that dances from the ever-flowing energy inside and around us. When there's an interference in our brain and nervous system, our innate or true potential cannot be expressed. My back pain was relieved first, but over time even more healing took place in my back and throughout my body. My cramps decreased, my headaches were eliminated, and my mental attitude began to turn around.

This is one of my favorite quotes, because my desire to help people encompasses humanity. It took me awhile to understand what Lao Tzu meant by this:

"If you want to awaken all of humanity, then awaken all of yourself, if you want to eliminate the suffering in the world, then eliminate all that is dark and negative in yourself. Truly, the greatest gift you have to give is that of your own self-transformation."

If you want to awaken all of humanity, then awaken yourself. Our "self" is physical, mental, and spiritual, encompassed in one being that is ever-flowing, producing continuous energy transmitting from above downward, inside outward connecting us to every living thing in the Universe. Now this starts to make sense why if we want to awaken all of humanity, then we must start first with ourselves. How could we possibly begin to help others if we are so dim on the inside, not ever having the capability of reaching our individual full potential?

Although I was under regular chiropractic care and believed in the power of the adjustment, I still had strong allopathic beliefs engrained in my brain, not having a full understanding of the power our body has to be able to heal itself. I continued to stay on the pill, putting artificial hormones in my growing, developing body, thinking I'll have to be on this until I want to try to have kids (which I may not even be able to have because of the endometriosis). Every year that went by, this notion continued to become engrained deeper and deeper into my belief system—below the line thinking—which became more prevalent than thinking positively.

With continuing to put chemicals in my body and having irritable bowel syndrome, negative beliefs that had accumulated since birth, when I was 19 years old my gynecologist found a lump in my breast. WHAT THE F*#@!? Freaked out and scared, I assumed the worst, especially with a family history of breast cancer and already having pre-cancerous cells on my cervix. It was a fibroid; thankfully not cancer, but it was still an abnormality. Even though I was under chiropractic care, it still matters what we put in our body, like when I was taking the Pill. It is still an artificial chemical, in addition to toxic stress, making the subluxations (misaligned vertebrae pinching on a nerve) in my spine that were already there worse.

Remember, everything is connected, so my brain's communication and innate healing to my breast tissue was interrupted with toxins from the pill, and any other toxin accumulated since birth, including the impact of negative daily thoughts. This set up the perfect environment for disease to fester and flourish. I also didn't start chiropractic care until I was 16 years old, so there was 16 years of damage, some of which is permanent. My subluxations first took place during my own birthing process, as do most cases. Subluxations can start while in the womb or from the birthing process, they are caused from any physical trauma, emotional stress or environmental toxin. This mainstream allopathic lifestyle is all too relatable. There are times when it is necessary to treat the body allopathically, and for that I am thankful. When it comes to genetics, we do have the ability to inhibit certain genes to be expressed like cancer genes, and so on. This all depends on lifestyle, environment, and mental thought.

When my paternal grandmother passed away, I was 10 years old. I remember wondering afterward why we are here and where we go after we die. I also remember feeling connected to something like a force or pull, but not understanding what it was. Just because you're told something doesn't mean it's true and just because you can't see something doesn't mean it's not there. Around early adolescence, I felt this connection even stronger. It was a beautiful, breezy 80-degree, sunny summer day in August in East Tawas, Michigan on Lake Huron. I was laying in the grass reading a book along with the breeze coming off the water. I could feel something greater than me and greater than all of us. At that moment, I just knew there was a higher power greater than any living thing on this planet and throughout the Universe. It was a feeling I had throughout my entire being, one of floating or dancing. It was the moment my conscious brain awakened with my spirit and I felt the power of our Divine Source. This brings me back to awakening our "self," this was my spiritual "self" waking up. Our Divine Source is always present, for me this is when my conscious brain connected with my spirit, another piece of the infinite dance.

Back to high school when I was still focused on becoming a surgeon, my chiropractor at the time, Dr. Kent Semlow, was not only helping me express my body's true potential by adjusting my spine, he also inspired me on the impact I could have with helping people improve their health, continue a healthy lifestyle, and help prevent them from ever needing most surgeries. I started working for him and two of his brothers, Dr. Ron and Dr. Bob, and I was able to see how far-reaching the chiropractic adjustment has on people. The transformation I saw in patients from when they walked in, even if they were there for maintenance adjustments, was astonishing. I could see their vibration, their power, become even brighter from when they first came in. This is when I knew I wanted to become a chiropractor.

Chiropractic College was incredibly fulfilling, solidifying the foundation for my passion scientifically, artistically, and philosophically. While in school, I took myself off the Pill, cleaning up my body and brain, and learned an adjustment to flip a tilted uterus. No more cramps or prescriptions! Once out of school, sharing my excitement of this new knowledge was incredibly challenging. Colleges have their hands tied for what the curriculum allows in the allotted time, leaving little opportunity to teach proper business procedures and education on communicating chiropractic clearly. So, you are left to figure it out, find a mentor or work for someone who hopefully knows what they are doing. Still feeling trapped inside, knowing there was something inside me wanting to be expressed, and continuing to go through life, making the most of it? There will always be highs and lows in life but it's our mindset, the happiness of our brain on how we choose to respond or react to the peaks and valleys. It is the difference between enjoying life or going through it saying, "Well, I guess this is how it's supposed to be."

About six years after becoming a chiropractor, a wife, and a mom of three boys, I still felt like there was something I was still searching for. I was at a continuing education seminar when I met Dr. Ed Plentz, a life coach in our chiropractic profession, the owner of The Plentz Academy of Chiropractic (The PAC), who taught me how to improve my communication skills, learn the tools and skills on running a successful business, and tools and strategies for overall self-improvement. This is where I found what I was searching for. This is when I woke up my mental health, my brain, and was finally able to communicate effectively my thoughts, my dreams my passion!

My own self-transformation continues in this ever-changing universal existence. Self-improvement is a way of life for me, and I found a way to do this by leaps and bounds at an event called The Ultimate Breakthrough Experience (UBE), an extension of The PAC. The title says it all; you are breaking through moments or thoughts stuck in our own mind, causing you to stay put and fear change instead of embracing it. I have been to several of these events and every time I discover something new about myself and peel away layers of fear. During this weekend, you are not only helping yourself, but you're helping all those who attend as well.

Listening to my intuition, I opened another door of opportunity when a close friend of mine, Dr. Helena Beacom invited me to learn another chiropractic technique, CATS (Cranial Adjusting Turner Style). Our cranial bones can move in the wrong position as early as the womb just like the vertebrae of the spine, from the birthing process or various types of head traumas.

Left uncorrected, these cranial bones will heal in the wrong position, causing an interference to the brain tissue, slowly turning off the communication link between neurons, causing a lack of blood flow, lack of nutrients, and toxins to build up in the areas of involvement, the same as what occurs with the spine. This stems from the birthing process or a variety of head traumas that can occur throughout life.

Shortly after learning cranial adjusting, I was then invited to a seminar of Dr. Terry Rondberg and Bryan Hixson to tie everything I had to offer into a way to test the health of our brain and body's cell function with The Brain Based Program. This is a baseline test to see the health of our body on a cellular level. This program is designed in order to maintain health and prevent chronic diseases later in life. I am now able to offer a whole body health and wellness program by testing the quality of your cells health, remove any interference on brain tissue and spinal nerves, continue to educate and inspire my patients effectively, offer advice on living a healthier lifestyle, offer a whole-food nutritional supplement that provides our daily requirements of fruits, vegetables and omegas that repair cellular damage all while getting back to trusting our body's ability to heal itself from the inside out. For all who are interested in breaking through fears and desire self-improvement are always welcome to The UBE Event. I am also becoming a coach myself to reach beyond my own community as to what chiropractic truly is, igniting the passion for those who are frustrated in practice as well as for students to know how to run a successful practice right from graduation.

We all have the ability inside us to overcome and replace negative beliefs that can hinder our purpose in this life's journey. Life is a journey of steppingstones, one leading to the next. Every step and every transformation can lead us in many directions with endless opportunities to maintain our self's harmony, like a flowing river. The knowledge and experiences we gain along the way prepare us for what's to come and how we respond or react is always our choice. With the knowledge you gain from this book, learn from it and take the action necessary to awaken yourself brighter, so you can get the most enjoyment out of every moment in life, which will have a positive effect on those around you. Through all the ebbs and flows, the healthier our mind, body, and spirit are, what we choose will give us greater peace on this Earth. You too can make a difference; you can do this by starting with yourself.

About the Author

Dr. Carly Sorrell

Dr. Sorrell is a graduate from Sherman College of Chiropractic and has practiced in Grand Rapids, Michigan for over 10 years. She has always had a passion for helping others further themselves since she was a little girl growing up in a suburb of Detroit. She has been able to fulfill her passion by guiding and educating her patients and their families on chiropractic care by removing the interference on the nervous system with the chiropractic adjustment, allowing their bodies to increase its internal healing ability to thrive and adapt to their environment with increased potential.

Dr. Sorrell also has a thirst for knowledge and over the last eight years has had the privilege to be mentored by Dr. Ed Plentz in business application, procedure administration, and overall self-improvement. She expanded her education with adding cranial adjustments, a brain-based program, and whole-food nutritional supplements to her practice. She has discovered a newfound passion for coaching from her own experiences and success with having a coach and is now helping those in her own profession through The PAC coaching program to discover their own successes. She is also a proud mother of three energetic boys who continue to bring an abundance of joy and welcomed challenges to her life every day.

Contact Information:
Chiropractic and Beyond
Telephone: (616) 322-4984
Email: Carlyfae77@yahoo.com

THE EYES HAVE IT!!

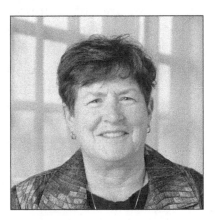

Dr. DeAnn M Fitzgerald, OD

"The real voyage of discovery consists, not in seeking new landscapes, but in having new eyes."
—Marcel Proust

In my perspective as an eye doctor, to be working at optimum brain activity, we must constantly check to "see" where the eyes are—both structurally and functionally. The eyes and vestibular system are intimately linked by a three-neuron system, with reflexive eye movements revealing how the brain is performing. As an example, the VOR (vestibular ocular reflex) allows the head and eyes to stay on target (i.e., observing telephone poles while driving along a road at rapid speed).

Vision is a multimodal activity of the brain and body:

- There are more than one million nerve fibers in each eye.
- Vision is the primary sense, with 40% of the cerebral cortex involved with processing visual information (i.e., making sense of what we see)

- 70% of our brain is dedicated to vision is some fashion
- 80% of all sensory input goes through our eyes
- 90% of people who have a concussion, traumatic brain injury, and stroke and/or neurodegenerative difficulty will have one or more visual affects
- 40% of those visual defects will be present even three months later if they are not addressed. If they are not addressed, it will also lead to delayed recovery.

Babies learn to see much like they learn to walk and talk. They must learn to use the visual information their eyes send to their brain in order to understand the world around them and interact with it appropriately. Vision, and how the brain uses visual information, are learned skills. We explore with our eyes. Even before babies reach and grab with their hands, crawl or sit up, they are looking around and taking in visual information. Therefore, providing visual information and stimulation are important for our development. What we really see is our mind's reconstruction of objects based on input provided by the eyes, not the actual light received by them. The eyes, directly or indirectly, are connected to the subcortex and total neurologic system, and vision emanates from the action system. The action system involves vision to support and organize proprioception, then to support posture, and finally to coordinate movement.

Our brain releases a chemical called BDNF (Brain Derived Neurotrophic Factor), which acts as a "fertilizer for the brain." When we move with a little higher intensity, this chemical is released. This is why movement is important for recovery and rehabilitation. By using vision, vestibular, auditory, and proprioception, we can 'boot' or 'reboot' our brain by using multi-modal systems.

Movement—Movement—Movement!

We are all moving less with today's amenities. Therefore, the lack of eye and body movement impacts the brain and brain function. The longer we sit, the more the brain shunts off blood and nutrients to certain areas. The eyes, as an extension of the brain, are no different.

When we sustain a concussion, TBI, stroke, or we begin to experience neurodegenerative decline, this causes the multimodal visual system to disconnect. The dorsal system (peripheral/motor) is fully myelinated at birth, the vestibular system is fully myelinated at birth, and then vision of the ventral system (central) connects with the nervous system three to six months later. Therefore, the last to join the system is in essence the first to disconnect when an insult compromises the nervous system. The result is that the dorsal, peripheral, and ventral/central system lose their ability to work efficiently together.

What does that mean?

It means that the balance and interaction between vision and motor function is compromised. Vision dysfunction causes recovery delays, interferes with learning, creates problems with communication, and affects memory by disrupting time and space, thus causing "focal binding." Focal binding compromises the preconscious/proactive relationship between the dorsal system (peripheral/motor), vestibular system, and proprioception. Movement becomes conscious (top down) and reduces function and fluency. There is no fluency because the system is no longer able to anticipate (i.e., reading, etc.).

Essentially, focal binding inhibits the release of detail, with the environment becoming overstimulated. In essence, these individuals can't see the forest for the trees. Movement in the environment (such as busy, crowded areas) becomes chaos to the visual system. Print on a page becomes a mass of detail, and movement of the eyes is projected into the field, causing movement of print or the perception of movement of the ground being walked on.

What is focal binding in neuro-terminology?

Hyper-action of the sympathetic nervous system occurs. This is the "fight or flight" response of pupil dilation, collapse of the peripheral visual system, with razor sharp acuity of the central visual pathway are compensatory responses.

Therefore, we don't even need to talk trauma. Fear reactions start in the brain and spread throughout the body, making adjustments for the best defense or flight reaction. The fear response starts in a region of the brain called the amygdala. This almond-shaped set of nuclei in the temporal lobe of the brain is dedicated to detecting the emotional salience of the stimuli, meaning how much something stands out to us.

For example, the amygdala activates whenever we see a human face with an emotion. This reaction is more pronounced with anger and fear. A threat stimulus, such as the sight of a predator, triggers a fear response in the amygdala, which activates areas involved in preparation for motor functions involved in fight or flight. It also triggers a release of stress hormones and the sympathetic nervous system. This leads to bodily changes that prepare us to be more efficient in response to danger. The brain becomes hyper-alert, pupils dilate, the bronchi dilate and breathing accelerates. Heart rate and blood pressure rise. Blood flow and a stream of glucose rush to the skeletal muscles. On the flip side of that coin, organs not vital in survival, such as the gastrointestinal system, slow down.

An area of the brain called the hippocampus is closely connected with the amygdala. The hippocampus and prefrontal cortex help the brain interpret a perceived threat. They are involved in a higher-level processing of context, which helps a person know whether a perceived threat is real. For instance, seeing a lion in the wild can trigger a strong fear reaction, but the response to a view of the same lion at a zoo is more of a curiosity. This is because the hippocampus and the frontal cortex process contextual information, and inhibitory pathways dampen the amygdala fear response and its downstream results. Basically, our thinking reassures our emotional areas of the brain that we are, in fact, okay. When our thinking brain gives feedback to our emotional brain, and we perceive ourselves as being in a safe space. We can quickly shift the way we experience high arousal states, going from one of fear to one of enjoyment.

The autonomic nervous system, also known as the involuntary nervous system, regulates those functions in the body that occur automatically, such as breathing, blood pressure, digestion, heartbeat, bladder function, and narrowing or widening of the blood vessels. It is composed of two branches, the parasympathetic nervous system and the sympathetic nervous system.

Sympathetic Nervous System

The sympathetic nervous system is also known as our stress response system, or the fight or flight system, and it is set into motion when we experience stress. It increases our heart rate and blood pressure, dilates pupils, restricts circulation, slows down digestion and urination, makes us more alert, providing a boost in energy so that we are capable of dealing with stressful situations effectively. It increases energy and is often referred to as the accelerator of the autonomic nervous system.

Parasympathetic Nervous System

The job of the parasympathetic nervous system is the exact opposite. Once the stressful event is over, it brings the heart rate and blood pressure back to normal, constricts pupils, improves circulation, enhances digestion, increases urination, calms us down, and puts us into a state of rest and relaxation. It conserves energy and is often referred to as the brakes of the autonomic nervous system.

Types of Stress on the Body

Emotional stress—This is the form of stress most people are familiar with and what comes to mind when they think of the term. This may include loss of any kind such as a divorce or breakup, loss of a job, loss of abilities or characteristics, depression, conflict in relationships, financial struggles, internal conflict, childhood abuse or neglect, dysfunctional or toxic relationships, employment issues, etc.

Cognitive stress—Unrealistic demands or expectations for yourself and/or your life, trying to live up to expectations of others, keeping up with the Joneses, seeing the glass half empty, catastrophizing, or awfulizing.

Sensory stress—Chronic pain, loud noise, or constant stimulation from external sources.

Metabolic stress—Syndrome X, too much exercise, pH, blood sugar issues, or hypoglycemia.

Toxic stress—I usually refer to this as environmental toxins. It includes things like heavy metal toxicity, amalgam fillings, mercury in your food, air pollution, electro smog, pesticides, herbicides, mold mycotoxins, disinfectants, perfume, air fresheners, etc.

Endocrine and neurotransmitter stress—Adrenal glands, cortisol, thyroid disorders, hormonal imbalances, menopause, andro-pause, insulin, dopamine, serotonin, norepinephrine, GABA, etc.

Purposelessness stress—I call this spiritual stress, characterized by a lack of meaning and purpose in life, inability to find gratitude, lack of love and empathy, not feeling connected to the Universe, or loss of self.

Infectious stress—Candida, parasites, viruses, bacteria, Lyme, etc.

Oxidative stress—Veins and arteries, emphysema, lack of fresh air, sleep apnea, Phase 1 and Phase 2 detoxification.

Energetic stress—Electromagnetic fields from cell phones, electronics, or geopathic stress.

Structural stress—Spine alignment, posture, TMJ, craniosacral, physical trauma, etc.

- If we have to devote attention to posture, we cannot attend to other things.
- Posture should be part of an organizational set that does not require conscious attention.
- If the sensorimotor system is out of balance, it will affect visual, cognitive and vestibular processing into anxiety and fear.
- Conversely, if visual processing is out of balance, it will affect sensorimotor, vestibular, and cognitive processing into anxiety and fear.

Priorities for Treatment:

1. **Double vision**—Lenses, prisms and multimodal therapies (brainstem).
2. **Light Sensitivity**—Tints, dynamic movement therapies (superior colliculus, basal ganglia).
3. **Vestibular problems**—Vision vestibular therapies (vestibular, brainstem, cerebellum)
4. **Focal/spatial imbalance**—Realigning dorsal/ventral system (frontal, parietal, temporal).
5. **Autonomic Nervous System**—Balancing sympathetic system and parasympathetic system (brainstem).

Treatment Strategies:

1. **Sleep**—We must get adequate sleep. Sleep hygiene, melatonin, amitriptyline, magnesium.
2. **Nutrition**—Autoimmune diet, paleo, Mediterranean, gluten/casein free.
3. **Pacing and planning**—Sub-symptomatic graded activity, ideas for non-provoking activities (audiobooks, podcasts).
4. **Headaches**—Medication, acupuncture, craniosacral, migraines, C-spine Treatment, BrainTap, syntonics, photo biomodulation.
5. **Noise sensitivity**—Musician filter ear plugs, graded exposure, Listening Program, dynamic movement therapies.
6. **Anxiety**—Mindfulness, meditation, craniosacral, easy movement, Tai Chi, breathing, gratitude journal.
7. **Using BrainTap for better sleep**—Work on decreasing anxiety and better balance for the sympathetic/parasympathetic system

Thoughts

If the proprioceptive system is not operating efficiently, the vestibular system is often affected. Tactile input has a large proprioceptive map; you can use this to your advantage in therapy. Therapy should target the integration of proprioceptive and vestibular systems for best results (high-tech equipment with eye-hand coordination tasks, such as Dynavision and Senaptec are great tools).

Problems Associated with Proprioception:

- Touch
- Balance
- Movement
- Decreased body awareness
- Stiffness
- Uncoordinated movement
- Clumsiness
- Falling
- Difficulty ascending and descending stairs
- Toe walking
- Slapping feet when walking
- Dyspraxia
- Difficulty with eating and speaking

Proprioception refers to sensory messages about the position, force, direction, and movement of our own body parts. Our muscles and joints assist us with "position sense." It sends messages about whether the muscles stretch or contract and how the joints bend and straighten. Gravity can stimulate the proprioceptive message without our conscious awareness. We have 25,000 proprioceptors in the feet, and vibration therapy is very effective for getting the brain to recognize feet.

A comprehensive "happy brain" approach has to include eyes and visual hygiene. If the National Football League and concussions have taught us anything, it's that lingering cognitive issues are really unresolved vision/vestibular issues. In addition, anxiety issues are ubiquitous. The limbic loop that creates anxiety can be altered by using vision/vestibular therapies. Also, cervical issues that remain are often unresolved vision/vestibular issues.

Essentially, eat a healthy diet with little sugar, caffeine and little alcohol. Get good sleep. Use your eyes, vestibular, balance and proprioception—you've got to move—create BDNF—take fish oils, Vitamin D3 and practice good breathing techniques.

1. Get your heart rate up.

Regular aerobic exercise boosts blood flow to the PFC (saccades) and has been shown to improve focus and impulse control. Aim for 30-45 minutes a day of fast walking (walk like you are late for an important appointment).

2. Eat a brain healthy diet.

Did you know that a sugar-filled junk food diet can fuel your addiction? Getting a quick sugar rush from soda, cookies, or candy weakens the PFC and can make you more impulsive. Eating lean protein throughout the day and eliminating sugar can help stabilize blood sugar levels, which is beneficial for your PFC, moods, and impulse control.

3. Supplement your diet.

Nutritional supplements, such as omega-3 fatty acids and green tea, just to name a few, that can boost blood flow to the PFC and help you stay focused on your goals.

4. Set goals for yourself.

Have great ambitions and high expectations for your life and your future. However, do not forget to remain grounded and humble. Be realistic about your life, while never letting go of your dream and your vision—and *make* a lot of joy!

"Keep your eyes on the stars, and your feet on the ground."

—Theodore Roosevelt

About the Author

Dr. DeAnn M Fitzgerald, OD

Practicing optometry since 1984 in Cedar Rapids, Iowa, Dr. Fitzgerald, began a 501c3 with Spanda Inc. "A single idea, a single action, can move the world." Beginning with Eyecare Kenya, bringing eyecare, medical care and water to a small village in Kenya, until political unrest prevented them from returning. In 2007, she opened a concussion, traumatic brain injury, and stroke clinic, providing baseline testing and proactive sports vision performance training to help hardwire the brain against neurodegeneration. No one, no matter what their economic resources, are turned away. Dr. Fitzgerald provides therapy for patients with cutting-edge ideas, providing "out of the box" treatment. "If not you, who? And if not now, when?"

Contact information:
Website: www.docfitzgerald.com
Telephone: 319-366-3500
Email: Drfitz4eyes@gmail.com
Address: 3225 Williams Parkway SW, Cedar Rapids, IA 52404

THE DREAM THAT CREATED MY DESTINY

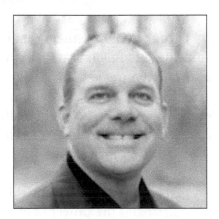

Dr. Ed Plentz

Imagine a four-year-old boy sitting across from his mother as she looks at him while strapped to a traction device saying, "Mommy is so sorry she hurts so bad," "Mommy is so sorry that she can't play with you," and, "Mommy is so sorry that …." She would proceed to pass out from the drugs and traction as the blue color left her face and arms. Traction relieved the pressure from her fractured neck as a result of an auto accident that didn't leave her paralyzed but caused extreme pain with migraines and neck pain. The surgeons did a fusion, that left her in flexion, and it cut the blood supply to her brain and arms.

That little boy was me. I would add weight to the traction device until I could see the color come back to her face, neck and arms. This literally freaked me out. My grandfather stated that we should take my mother to a chiropractor as they can't hurt her because she already had a fractured neck. The next thing you know, we were heading an hour north to Michigan to go see this chiropractor as a last resort.

We lived in Ohio at the time and you couldn't go to a chiropractor back then because of the scope of practice in Ohio. You see, a person couldn't go to a chiropractor in Ohio at the time because they classified it as practicing medicine without the proper license. That meant we had to drive to Michigan to get my mother's power turned back on. Now remember, this was the early 70s and Michigan had the best scope laws in our profession back then.

Even though I tried to convince them that I could stay home by myself, my family did not buy it and I had to make the trek to Michigan to this so-called miracle man to help my mother. (Side note: as a grown man I shouldn't be left alone too long because I'm like a hummingbird with a turbo charger attached to it, and I can and still will get into a ton of trouble if I'm left alone to long.) So, it was a very wise call on my parents' part about not letting me stay home.

I'm very happy that I did make those long rides up to Michigan and that I got to see firsthand the power of chiropractic as I had witnessed my mother become human again. It was just amazing, and I became very curious and intrigued at a very young age about this profession that saved my mother's life. Fast-forward to four years later. I'm now eight years old and I have seen my mother get adjusted many times. Though I never experienced an adjustment yet, I did see many other miracles happening in this doctor's office.

Then "IT" happened, the dream that created my destiny, the calling that woke me up to my life's quest to where I am today. I remember it like it was yesterday. I ran down the steps full of excitement as I anxiously told my family that I was going to be a "Crack-o-Practor" one day. I couldn't even pronounce the name right. They laughed and I became focused. I shared my enthusiasm with the doctor in Michigan and he gave me a job to clean his office. That doctor retired and the new doctor aka "Doc," became my new mentor and guide on my hero's quest. I went to seminars with him at age 12. I then delved into the philosophy of chiropractic and the "why" behind this wonderful profession. By the time I went to Palmer Chiropractic College in

Davenport, Iowa, I had already had 15 years of experience and study in our profession (from age 4 to age 19), when I enrolled at Palmer. I knew the "why" of chiropractic, but I didn't know the "how."

I loved school and devoured any information on science, technique, philosophy, the practical application of business, and patient education. This was done with only one purpose in mind: to get out of school and serve as many people in my community that I could so they and their families could be healthier naturally. It was in October of 1991 that I graduated, and with degree in hand and on a whim and a prayer, I opened my first clinic in January of 1992. I just knew I was going to be successful, but the Universe had a different plan. I grew somewhat, but I was just paying my bills. I was located in a town of 1,100 with two other chiropractors. I started to think that maybe this town just didn't get me, chiropractic, or anything else that came out of my mouth for that matter. I had this passion, this life song, that started to fade as I realized that though I may sing great in the shower per se, my patients and community didn't hear my song, as I must have stunk singing onstage. But I didn't give up. I knew people needed to be adjusted, sick or well, to keep that vital connection from the brain to the body open and free of interference.

I started to search for help and three years into practice, I found just that. I met a man named Dr. Joseph Flesia. He took a liking to me and he was a pioneer, an icon, and one charismatic leader in our profession. He showed me how to communicate, educate, and inspire my patients and my community about the wonders of chiropractic instead of marketing, selling and closing them on a healthcare service. He taught me how to speak their language so my community embraced chiropractic as a lifestyle, opposed to a symptom relief procedure. He showed me how to sing great on stage so that my passionate song could be heard everywhere I went, and boy oh boy, I started signing! My practice exploded from 150 patient visits a week to over 200 each day. I was really living my dream and helping many others be healthy by allowing them to experience a healthy brain and nervous system.

This success in my clinic and my relationship with Dr. Joe

led me to speaking platforms around the world. I was telling my story and teaching these communication technologies to all who would listen and learn so they could make their communities a better place to live by increasing the health levels of all the people who lived there. "Healthier People = Healthier Planet" became my mantra. I purchased Dr. Joe's company with a business partner and that led us to spreading the word to thousands of DCs worldwide. Recently after 20-plus years my business partner and I parted ways and I started a new company called The PAC—a/k/a Plentz Academy of Chiropractic—that is dedicated to the same vision but is a supercharged version of my previous company I was involved in. It is amazing how using hindsight as a 20/20 gauge of how much you can improve things from that line of experience. The PAC's vision is to show every DC and DC2B (Doctor of Chiropractic to be) on the planet how to communicate, educate, and inspire every man, woman, and child on the importance of the chiropractic lifestyle's healthcare regime.

It has been one fantastic ride, for sure. Our student program focuses on the DC2B and prepares them from day one of school of how to sing that song right upon graduation, so they become successful right from the start. Our doctors' program is designed to take an existing office that has maybe been missing its mark and not seeing the patients they expected, making them the most sought-after chiropractor in their community.

How do we do this? We get you involved, we show you our proven patient educational plan, and then you enjoy your dream practice. It doesn't do you or the planet any good if you don't have patients on your tables. They want what we have; we just have to communicate it in way that they can see, hear, and feel it like we do. We will show you that plan and help you either start right from the beginning, having the right procedures, or show you how to implement them in your existing office to help your practice grow predictably. The result of all of this is more people experiencing the miracles of chiropractic on a wellness level. It is you as the doctor feeling great about your profession and keeping your passion fueled for years of faithful service to your community and profession. Most importantly though is allowing the potential of each and every patient who enters your office the ability to be their best because their brain and nervous system are as healthy as they can be.

We all know the importance of having a healthy brain and nervous system, but the general public doesn't. They are educated on chasing symptoms and not interested unless taught how to increase health, so their symptoms disappear instead of hiding them with drugs or surgery. They are in an "outside in, below upward" approach instead of an "above down, inside out" mentality which is the Chiropractic way and philosophy of health. Look at it this way. If a person is put on blood pressure medication, they are doing nothing for heart health they are just participating in symptom suppression. What do I mean by this? The blood pressure drug just lowers the blood pressure artificially, but it isn't doing anything to make the heart healthier. We know this because if you take the drug away, their blood pressure goes right back up.

How about a different approach? How about addressing the main stresses on our bodies and showing our patients how to be healthier as a whole so that their cells, organs, systems, and bodies all become healthier and function better? We address this with them with a three-prong approach of thoughts, traumas and toxins. With thoughts, we address their mental attitude and create an environment of health and excitement for them and their families. We show them to be "above the line" thinkers instead of "below the line," negative thinking like most of society. We address their traumas and structural issues of their brain and nervous system through regular chiropractic adjustments for themselves and their families. This will give them the best chance to function at a higher level of health as the brain and nervous system controls and coordinates every function of our body. We address toxins in their systems through whole food nutrition. We want ourselves and our patients to have the proper fuel to be the best that they can be and to be able to function at the highest level they possibly can. Exciting isn't it? If everyone knew the importance of chiropractic care as a lifestyle, this world would be a better place.

What happens if we don't do this? Well, the writing is on

the wall. Just read the headlines in the papers and on the web. Are we as a species getting healthier or sicker? Our children are consuming a huge number of drugs at a very young age and it's the first time in our existence that it is predicted adults will outlive their children. Can you believe that? I can't, and I won't accept it either. We must communicate, educate, and inspire all those we come into contact with and show them that there is a different way for them to take care of themselves and their family. That their body is incredible, and when there is no interference, it can do incredible things.

Think about it. Your body built you from two tiny little cells and nine months later, you came into this world. All 10 fingers and 10 toes, your lungs in the right place, your heart beating automatically, food eaten, and waste eliminated, eyes that see and don't smell, ears that hear and don't see, and this power in the body has built other bodies perfectly for eons of time. Do you think this power that has done all of this but forgot to put in an immune system or how to adapt to the environment around it? I think not.

How do you think it would be if everyone had a healthy brain and nervous system? There would be less aches and pains, fewer drugs consumed, fewer surgeries performed, and more people expressing their inner potential at a higher level than ever imagined. They would be able to be a better version of themselves and express that in their jobs, hobbies, and families. There would be less crime and illnesses, and the world would be a happier, healthier place to live.

You see, a healthier brain and nervous system is a must if you want to be your best. It is our fundamental operating system that controls every single function in our body and we only get one, so we had better learn how to take care of it or we are going to have problems.

The PAC's specialty is doing just that, giving you the DC2B or the chiropractor in the field the strategies, procedures and patient educational tools to educate every single person that comes through your door about the importance of having a healthy brain and nervous system, as well as their family having a healthy brain and nervous system from birth to death. If you would like to learn more how to do this in your practice, you can contact us at the addresses listed below.

We have one purpose as chiropractors on this planet in my opinion, and that is to teach and serve as many people as we can on how to take care of their brain and nervous system so they can be their healthiest. Does one person make a difference? You bet you do! Everyone you touch and everyone you serve is different after they leave your office than when they entered. By adjusting them, you are allowing "The power that has made the body, which is the power of perfection" to express itself 100% and once that is done, all that can be done has been done. Now go and share your message, express your passion, and change the planet one spine at a time.

About the Author

Dr. Ed Plentz

"Dr. Ed" as many know him by, has been in practice and a pillar within the business community of the famous Brooklyn/Irish Hills area of Michigan for over 25 years. Dr. Ed has provided the highest quality of chiropractic care to patients ranging from newborns to great-grandparents, athletes, to service members and everyone in between. In and out of the office, he emphasizes "wellness" care over sick care. He has been a consultant to thousands of doctors around the world, so they can bring this same quality of wellness care to their communities.

Dr. Ed is an international author, the founder of the Plentz Academy of Chiropractic (The PAC), and lecturer for numerous groups and professional organizations. Additionally, he is a proud board member of the World Chiropractic Alliance. Dr. Ed is a husband of 24 years to Angela, a proud father to three beautiful daughters, Summer, Jordan, and Jasmin, and soon-to-be grandpa to two beautiful babies.

Contact Information:
Website: www.plentzacademyofchiropractic.com
Email: eplentz@comcast.net

YOU DON'T NEED TO ENDURE SICKNESS TO HAVE AN EPIPHANY

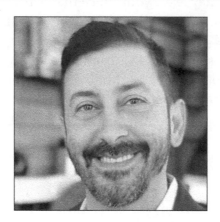

Dr. Guillermo Barquet

A lot of people around my age have a wakeup call almost for the exact same reasons: an illness, a disease, or a loss. As for me, it was God's way of telling me to shut up for just one moment.

In the year 2005, I was 26 at the time, and my stomach couldn't take it anymore. For years, my gastritis developed into an ulcer, and I promise you, it felt like an erupting volcano inside me. As a dental surgeon, I knew that the proton pump inside my stomach was producing too much acid to the point that was unbearable. What no one taught me at school is that anger, rage, and frustration were the real causes of all that lava erupting and erosion in my esophagus.

That night the pain was so excruciating that my dad drove me to the hospital. The diagnosis after having an endoscopy performed hit me like an asteroid at a million miles per hour. A polyp. A type of cancer. And conveniently located in the middle of a vocal cord.

It took two surgeries on my throat and stomach in 10 days (in addition to a fractured upper maxillary during the first procedure). The anesthesiologist was so unprofessional with my care that he just cracked my bone, losing four teeth in the process. I was devastated. The good news in all this chaos was that the lab results of the polyp came back benign, and the nerve in my vocal cord remained intact. I feared more the loss of my voice than having to endure chemo or radiation. Being an introvert in my early years, I was just learning to communicate with my fellow humans. In a snap, I was told before entering the operating room that there was a big risk of losing my ability to speak.

It took me days to actually understand the words of my surgeon: "The problem you showed up with is seen in people above 65, not at your age. I emphatically recommend you look for alternative medicine. Something different. Don't stick only to medication."

My first encounter with something other than synthetic drugs was biofeedback and my mind exploded. It was so amazing, refreshing and exciting how the session revealed the *real* me. I learned how I had to develop this annoying, egomaniac, smarty-pants, arrogant, dumbass personality, and it was just a cover—a defense mechanism, pure and simple. At that moment, I despised myself, my life, my parents, my past, and all the things that made me what I had become. In the end, learned that I was afraid.

A few months after my first biofeedback session, I was so hooked up that I sold every single dentistry instrument. Everything in the dental clinic was out the door in a couple of days, and after burning the bridge (which I didn't understand until recently), I bought my first device and started a whole new approach to life. To my life. I became one of the most successful and recognized biofeedback practitioners in my country. I started giving courses and lectures, doing sessions in different cities in Mexico and overseas. I also found a way of seeing 12 clients a day, achieving outstanding results. My stubbornness paid off and I was on a roll.

But then, the fear came back.

That damned sensation.

It appeared after my son was born.

Our pregnancy was beautiful, amazing, and so full of joy for me and my wife. Antonio was for sure the most expected baby in the Universe! He is all we could ever imagine, with just an itty-bitty detail: he had developed a hiatal hernia, just like his daddy. His first couple of months were very difficult for us, trying too much and too hard to help his condition, and we worried every time he vomited. I saw him grow, but just his little bones. He was a small, weightless little thing. My worries became anger, comparing the results I had at my clinic. I had overcome an illness, along with countless people, too. Even one lady with a kidney transplant failure came out of a sure death, and this baby boy, my primary concern in life, didn't respond to my methods. My conflicted heart splattered on the floor when our pediatrician in threw the towel in the most painful and conscious way. "I can't do more for you guys. You need to find a gastric pediatrician because this is getting out of hand."

We found one, made an appointment, and up we went. He was wonderful! My wife had to make major changes to her diet (taking food away from any lady makes her the most irritable person alive). Something the doctor said hit me like a hammer. Catecholamine, a neurotransmitter from the sympathetic nervous system, were flooding mommy's milk, damaging the inner lining of Antonio's stomach. Stress! Oh... my... God!

At that time, continuing my search for something else to help my son, the same person that introduced me to biofeedback gave me my first LED light therapy device. I was extremely skeptical. How can a neoprene pad full of red and infrared diodes do more than a computerized system focused on stress reduction? I know I needed a miracle, but my narrowed mind was still confused. By just "turning it on and putting it on," the LEDs delivered. In less than a month, Antonio stopped all of his tummy meds and started gaining weight. BAM! Mind blown! How could this be?

Light therapy, or chromotherapy, is as old as any other medicine and has been practiced since 2000 B.C. in Egypt, Greece, China, and India. People in that age didn't understand the medical concepts of light but had faith in the restorative process of the body through color. Light is energy, and the phenomenon of color is just the interaction between energy and matter. All our organs, cells and atoms exist as energy, and each part of us has a frequency or vibrational energy. Each of our organs and energy centers vibrate and harmonize with the frequencies of colors. When various parts of the body deviate from these expected normal vibrations, we can assume that the body is either diseased or at least not functioning properly. The vibratory rates inherent in the vibrational technique (chromotherapy) are such that they balance the diseased energy pattern found in the body. For in every organ, there is an energetic level at which the organ functions best. Any departure from that vibratory rate results in pathology, whereas restoring the appropriate energy levels to the physical organs results in a healed body.

My brain is still on the floor by learning these things. I now know how my son's body reacted so perfectly to the stimulation of LEDs. He activated his self-healing capabilities through light stimulation, and he recovered.

In addition to the person who gave me the light device, I was invited to México City to help with a series of conferences focused on quantum/biofeedback practitioners and what do you know? The owners of the company who fabricate the LED device I had at home were also in attendance. I met this impressive couple, and after dinner the lady asked, "What do you see yourself doing in the next few years?" I don't know if she was being polite, but I took the question seriously, and in three seconds I blurted, "Working for a company like yours!"

Well, that was all it took. We started exchanging emails and phone calls, and before I knew what was happening, they invited me to California. I now know this was my last test. We had a chat to cover minor details and they embraced me like family. I started to work in the medical staff of a company made from scratch in their garage, founded with love, with one thing in mind: let the world know that light therapy works.

Those three years were the best education I could ever have. I felt real love outside my family. I busted my ass traveling, learning, teaching, and spreading the word. I met amazing people, visionaries, and experts in numerous fields. Because of this, my understanding of the word healing took another dimension. Photons, which is the quantum unit of energy, can penetrate the skull, restoring blood flow to the brain, aiding in the production of neurotransmitters, regulating anti-social behavior, unexplained anger, and sudden changes in mood. Neurorehabilitation is clinically proven, and medical studies supported it. It is impossible not to think of the repercussion this could have in myself or any other human being.

I can control my emotions by just delivering light therapy to my head. I can restore my sleeping patterns to an almost normal state by just allowing unrestricted blood flow to my brain. I can help people with a concussion or with post-traumatic stress. But this is the most incredible part: we were taught in medical school that the only tissue that cannot regenerate is neurons. It had been a mantra of biology that brain cells do not regenerate. In a startling scientific discovery made in the late 1990s, researchers at Princeton University found that new neurons were continually being added to the brains of adult monkeys. Up until recently, more and more studies suggest that the human brain can restore itself.

Physical and emotional trauma can have a huge effect in our behavior. PTSD is something you cannot see, but any person suffering from it can feel it. These symptoms are so powerful that people can commit suicide. The sun is an exceptional source of healing light. There are many places where you can find light therapy devices, and there are some very cheap choices on the Internet. All you need is a reason to do something for yourself. This can save your life; it can save all our lives.

So, keep in mind we are learning how to have a happy brain. We need to be emotionally stable. All I need to be the greatest human being is to have emotional health.

I teach my patients every day about controlling emotions, I have seen people in mental shock after losing someone or enduring a financial breakdown, or a divorce. The first thing we all have to do after any trauma is to practice gratitude. The one thing between you and emotional health is your ego. Being grateful is the best medicine, and the best thing is that you don't need to go to school, attend a seminar, or take a course to learn gratitude. You only need to close your eyes, take a deep, deep breath, and say it in your mind: I'm grateful! I have a personal mantra that I hope can help you. Repeat after me:

"I will speak great things into existence for my life. I know the power of my mind. I know the power of my words. I'll use my innate powers to consciously change my reality. Everything starts with me."

I wrote many articles in the best newspaper in my hometown, and they all have to do with things I teach to my patients at the clinic. Here are some tips for a happy brain and emotional health:

1. **Every person is happy in their own way.**

Try not to impose your thinking or methods on your loved ones. Every mind and personality are different, even your children. Guide them, learn from them, and stop yelling to them. Just LISTEN!

2. **Water will never boil if we pay too much attention to it.**

Problems won't go away if you think too much about them. Focus your mind on the outcome, not in the journey.

3. **Love is really, really simple.**

It's very easy to not lie, to not disappoint, and to be there. Do for your partner what you think your mom would do with you.

4. **Digital dementia.**

Pay close attention to your posture. Looking at your computer or cellphone with a tilted head might impede oxygen to the brain, causing all kinds of neural disorders.

5. **If today I have you, I cherish you.**

This is something we all see in movies, so every time you see the words live, laugh, love, eat, sleep, and many more, put them into practice. Focus on living like there's no tomorrow. Live one day at a time, one hour at a time.

5a. If today I don't have you, I'm grateful.

Instead of crying all day, thinking of what could have happened or what you didn't or couldn't do, take a massive breath and say out loud, "Thank you! Thank you for everything! All the time, adventures, and moments, I cherish them completely." You'll see that the pressure on your chest will decrease dramatically as the hours go by.

6. You are the sun of your own solar system.

Your energy is limited. Compare it to a full tank of gas; if you don't plan in advance, or drive recklessly, you will waste your fuel unnecessarily. Think before throwing away your energy on things that don't matter to you. You come first, always.

7. If your partner is an apple tree and you are a pear tree, why would you expect to be equals?

Don't try to change what a person is. If the apple tree that you chose only gives 10 apples a year and three feet of shadow, but you expect it to change as the relationship goes by, you will be disappointed. Try to pull it so it can grow, and you will snap it. Don't push your partner to be like you or try to change their essence or push too hard for him or her to grow. Sometimes 10 apples are all they can offer. If that is not enough for you, then you are the one who must change.

8. Does luck exist?

Every small thing you do for yourself or other people has a direct impact in the world. Do good, and good will come back. Give, and you will be given. Forgive, forget and let go, and you make space for new and wonderful things to grow in you. For me, that's luck.

9. You are not Superman.

It makes no sense to be available for other people, help them, and worry about them if you need help yourself. Until you are happy with yourself and have control of your habits, you cannot be there for someone else. You come first, then take on the rest.

10. Emotions do hurt, mentally and physically.

Every thought creates an emotion, and every emotion has a direct impact on our body. Think positive, and that will make you feel positive, thus your body recovers. Do it the other way around and see for yourself how your physical plane gets interrupted and pain/inflammation/illness will become present. Change how you feel by having great thoughts!

11. I am a black belt at controlling emotions.

Every time you encounter any problems and learn from them, you become an expert in that specific area. It's impossible to learn new things and not grow. As I see it, every time you face a challenge and overcome it, you master new ways. As in Karate, you advance in belt colors because you are getting better than the day before. When you realize that your energy is the most valuable asset in the Universe and stop wasting it on trivialities and stupidities, you will become a master.

I read somewhere about the analogy of the glass of water in your hand. Think about it for a moment. If you hold it high for a minute, it's not a problem. But as time passes, you'll have an ache in your arm, then it will feel numb or paralyzed. The weight of the glass doesn't change, but the longer you hold it, the heavier it becomes. That is exactly how stress and worry affect us. Think about it for a while and nothing happens. Keep thinking about it and it will start to hurt. Think about them all day long and you will feel numb and paralyzed, incapable of doing anything.

Put the glass down as quickly as you can.

About the Author

Dr. Guillermo Barquet

Dr. Guillermo Barquet was invited to be a speaker at the 4th Annual Brain Injury Conference in Colorado, did a presentation inside an NFL team, briefly helping some players to have a fast physical and mental recovery, and worked closely with military war veterans, focusing on the treatment of PTSD. He worked with a Mexican League baseball team as part of the medical staff giving onsite therapies to players before and during games. He was involved in the medical analysis of a clinical trial in a hospital in the US, using light therapy to accelerate healing in open wounds. Dr. Barquet is an international bilingual speaker, lecturing on LED therapy and its many applications in the US, Mexico, and Canada. He has a full-time clinic that helps clients with stress management and fast physical recovery using Biofeedback and LED light therapy.

Contact Information:
Email: memobarquet@gmail.com
Instagram: @guillermobarquet
Facebook: Guillermo Barquet
Phone number / WhatsApp: +5218441626529

HEALTH COMES FROM WITHIN

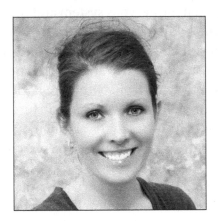

Dr. Helena Beacom

I am a wife and mother, but I was first a chiropractor. This is my story and how I became the chiropractor I am today. This is how and why I have the passion to help mothers like myself and their children. It is because of my children that I do what I do. I hope my story lets you know that you are not alone, and that even when MDs tell you they are out of answers, there is one more that you haven't tried and one that will change your life if you are brave enough to do something different.

I have been on a health journey for nearly two thirds of my life. I have been fortunate to find mentors at different stages of this journey to guide me through the unknown. Each step allows me to better care for my pediatric practice members as well as my own children, and for that I am extremely grateful.

As a kid, I had a lazy eye, suffered from chronic ear infections, and needed help with speech in elementary school. I had cranial nerve damage and spinal nerve damage from the process of childbirth that I wasn't even aware of. After 15 years of antibiotics, my immune system gave up on me and I suffered from yet another ear infection, tonsillitis, and bronchitis, which took me months to fight off. This was when I started to learn about chiropractic. I discovered a way to take care of myself without drugs or surgery. During my first three years under chiropractic care, I wasn't sick once. No common cold, no bronchitis, and finally, no more *ear infections*. With my first chiropractor, I started to *experience* the connection between the nervous system and the immune system. I learned that the body wants to be healthy and has everything inside it to do just that. I realized that the body can heal itself as long as you consistently remove any interference to that healing. I learned that health starts from within, regardless of what you're diagnosed with or suffer from. I went to chiropractic school to continue my journey of learning about natural health, but it took having my own children to really search and stretch my understanding of this topic.

I wanted to have my children born at home. Statistically, up to 80 percent of babies born vaginally at a hospital suffer from birth trauma to the head and neck. A C-section guarantees damage to the head and neck, which explains why I suffered so much as a child.

My husband and I opted to work with local midwives to attend to our children's births. We are fortunate to have beautiful, talented, dedicated, and experienced midwives here in West Michigan. Unfortunately, my water broke two days early and I stopped progressing hours into labor. The decision was made by the midwives to transfer us to a nearby hospital. In order for this hospital to accept me, I had to agree to an antibiotic IV. I still managed to have a natural birth at the hospital, but it was assumed that I had Group B strep, although testing never confirmed this. My baby was put on an IV antibiotic and we were threatened with CPS if we didn't stay in the hospital for 10 days. As a result of the antibiotics, we noticed our little girl's body would randomly jump out of control. The negative effect the antibiotics had on her nervous system was horrendous. We were very diligent about her chiropractic adjustments to aid in healing and take the pressure off of her nervous system. It took six months of regular chiropractic adjustments for her body to heal from the damage caused by the antibiotics.

Due to the experience I had in the hospital, I was determined to have our second child at home. This time I wanted to know the feeling of having my baby in my own bed. I had a beautiful birth experience with our son. I sat in the birthing tub for 45 minutes after he was born, just holding and looking at this amazing little boy in my arms. After the umbilical cord stopped pulsating, my husband cut it, then wrapped our son in a blanket and gave him his first chiropractic adjustment. Even in a healthy, truly natural birth, there can be interference to the delicate nerves in a newborn's neck. The picture of our son's first adjustment is in his first-year scrapbook as a very important occasion.

After the birth, I climbed into bed with our baby and lay with him all day and all night long. Do you remember that moment; that newborn smell? Holding your new baby in your arms for the first time? Snuggling with them that first night? As beautiful as that moment was, I couldn't get him to nurse. I tried for almost two weeks. I kept in contact with my midwives, but the pain was excruciating. I would cry before attempting to get him to latch, but I would do it anyway because it was that important to me. At his two-week checkup, it was determined that our son was tongue-tied. He was literally chewing me and getting very little breast milk. I was relieved to have an answer, yet I was horrified. Our son had to have his tongue surgically cut and he started to nurse immediately. He started to put on weight and my heavy heart became lighter.

Our son was finally eating and growing. When he started sitting up on his own, I put him in the bathtub and realized his head was very asymmetrical in shape. I didn't like what I saw, but I didn't know what to do about it either and it bothered me. Our son started rolling at five months old, but then stopped. He didn't start again until he was nine months old. At 11 months, our son started doing the army crawl. Between rolling and the army crawl, he could get anywhere. He would put his butt in the air, trying to establish a "normal" crawl, but to no avail. My husband and I adjusted his spine consistently, but his slow progress bothered us. We felt there was something we were missing but didn't know how to address his asymmetrical skull bones.

Every parent's worst nightmare is when they turn their back

and their child falls. In fact, it is estimated that 50% of children fall from a high place. It happens in a heartbeat and is heart wrenching. I had put him down in the middle of our bed for a moment and heard the worst sound I ever heard: a thump and then his cry. Our son stopped nursing and went back to chewing. I had to resort to pumping to get him the breastmilk he needed. When a mother desperately wants to nurse their baby, but for various reasons baby doesn't want to nurse, it is really hard emotionally for her. I didn't understand brain function to the degree that I do now, and I definitely didn't understand how to properly help or adjust my son's cranial/skull bones with the damage that ensued after his fall. I didn't know his fall interfered with the cranial nerve that supplies the tongue and allows it to move properly. Even though the tongue tie was cut, there is a neurological tie at the back of the head can interfere with a baby being able to nurse properly.

At our son's first birthday, there was a little boy who was younger than him, yet much more physically advanced. This little guy could go from sitting, to his belly, to crawling, and to sitting in a heartbeat. Our son could only sit or lay on his belly if you put him there, but he had no ability to change positions by himself. Our son was still not crawling normally, cruising, or walking. If I tried to hold his hands to get him to walk, his legs were straight and would not bend. Our son could not jump.

When our son was 13 months old, I saw a friend at a chiropractic seminar in Detroit. Dr. Karen Barsness, DC was trained to work on cranial/skull misalignments. She adjusted him multiple times that day. When we got home, we sat him on the floor to play. For the first time, he looked up to see what was on the couch and he started to cruise along furniture within 24 hours of his cranial adjustments. A month later, he climbed up an entire flight of stairs while his big sister encouraged him from the top. He did a lot more sign language than actual words, but he was communicating.

Because I couldn't find a cranial practitioner in West Michigan, I started to study under Dr. Roger Turner, DC in October 2012. Our son started making great progress, but he still wasn't walking or talking much. I decided to take him to Dr.

Turner in April 2013. At this point, he was 22 months old but still not walking. I had to hand him over to someone I trusted. I was too emotionally connected to what our son was or was not doing and couldn't think straight. Dr. Turner worked on our son for three straight days, four to five adjustments per day, performing adjustments to his head and spine. On day three, our son turned suddenly and walked from a chair to a table. At 22 months old, he finally walked on his own! By the time we left Dr. Turner's office, he was taking eight steps. I drove from Dr. Turner's office in Toronto to Detroit to have our son walk to his dad for the first time. With friends and family around, it was extremely emotional.

After seeing Dr. Turner, our son was standing on his own and walking. He would now walk and "right" himself and keep walking. Our son took more and more steps every day. He was trying more words on his own and doing more sign language. I followed Dr. Turner all over the place, from Toronto, to Chicago, to St. Lucia, so I could continue to study. The more I continued to learn about brain and nervous system function, the more people I could help.

I believe the chemical, emotional, and physical stress on our children has its effects generationally. Even with natural births, I see skull bones that don't return to their normal shape, putting so much pressure on different areas of the brain. More and more children have misshapen skulls that interfere with the cranial nerves in the brain. This interference is seen in the baby's inability to latch, nurse successfully, and develop properly, especially through the first year. It can be seen later with issues in speech, reading, and writing. Children have amazing results with cranial and spinal care. Creating positive change to the body takes time. Health is a lifelong journey; it is not a quick fix. Creating and maintaining health begins with both brain and nervous system function, and it has become my lifelong mission for myself, my children, and our community.

I can say that my passion lies with helping those babies with asymmetrically shaped heads or children that have developmental delays from growth to walking, to speech, and that is true. However, I am extremely passionate about decreasing the stress on mothers. I know how it feels to have a child not doing what your heart says they should be able to do. I know how it feels to be lost and without answers. I know how it feels to not know where to turn. I know how it feels, and I have been there at different times in my life.

Our son is making amazing progress every day. He works so hard in school, and physically, you would never know he had taken so long to crawl, cruise, walk, or speak. At the bottom of every developmental problem is the need for better nervous system and brain function. I am here for you and your children. I want to share everything I have learned. Your children deserve to get the help they so desperately need.

About the Author

Dr. Helena Beacom

Dr. Beacom is a chiropractor in Whitehall, Michigan. She has been passionate about helping infants and children since she graduated Palmer College of Chiropractic in 2002. Dr. Helena is dedicated to making a change to the health potential and future of our youths. You can find Dr. Helena spending time with her children, helping others' children, in her garden, or by the lakeshore.

Contact Information:
Beacom Family Chiropractic
923 E. Colby St.
Whitehall, MI 49461
231-893-1744
www.beacomchiro.com

EMPOWERING YOUR HAPPY BRAIN

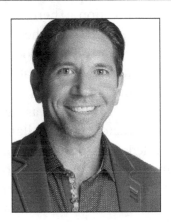

Dr. Jared A Leon

Imagine waking up one day as a young teen in a hospital bed with a multitude of severe injuries, in pain and not remembering how you got there? The poignant smells of a hospital, the beeping sounds of a ventilator and heart monitors, tubes everywhere, and the feeling of not being able to get up are exactly what occurred to myself when I was 14 years old on that grim, life-changing Labor Day. Many months of an arduous hospital journey followed by several years of further surgeries and healing created a perfect storm leading to a "why me" complex and darkened spirit.

Innately knowing this was not the reason for my survival from the horrific car accident that day, my newer, more enlightened self started to emerge. This turned into my own internal battle with some really big questions as a young man and forged a yearning to become a healer as a physician and my journey into medical school. A slight detour and blow to my ego occurred as I was deferred from medical school, and a feeling of despair and depression swept over me. Knowing that I still believed in the process of becoming a doctor and that perseverance became my mantra, a random idea and opportunity showed up that would change the course of my life.

I fully intended to carry out my childhood dream of becoming a medical doctor and applied to both medical and chiropractic schools, as the credits from the latter would ultimately transfer. So, my journey to Life Chiropractic University in Marietta, Georgia was my new direction. There, I was presented with amazing information about the true healing of the body and how the nervous system controls and coordinates every cell in the body. If something interferes with that signal, healing will be affected. Learning this concept changed everything, and on the fourth day of chiropractic school, I was determined to pursue a profession as a chiropractor, not an allopath. Unlike my past recovery that was filled with surgeries, medications, various therapies, and a team of doctors and nurses that barely explained anything to me (let alone why or how these symptoms have and kept affecting me), this gentle idea of innate wisdom was the spark I needed to find my true purpose.

My chiropractic mission was well on its way and four years of intense training and studying led me on the path to further healing, inspiring me to become a true healer. Feeling so blessed for the opportunity, I was a sponge to all things that could help people to heal, from various chiropractic techniques and certifications, to practicing anywhere and everywhere to better understand how to find and correct spinal misalignments and neurological interference.

Fast-forward a decade and being in private practice pragmatically getting good results with functional chiropractic, life was good, but I still felt another urge to push the boundaries and grow. With the erudite within starting to push outwards, I started my next chapter of my neurological enlightenment by starting a two-year rigorous functional neurology program and an additional vestibular rehabilitation fellowship. This material was like the Holy Grail that truly helped me to understand the inner workings of the human brain and how to apply this knowledge to rehabilitate and unlock the brain's true potential of healing. With an almost infinite amount of information to study and learn, I was humbled by the knowledge and the privilege to wield it as my healing weapon.

While homing in on my senses and amplifying my ability to observe my patients, I started to really see how the big picture of healing can be applied by the most gentle and slight inputs to the nervous system could have such a great impact on a person's life force. It was inspiring! For example, I was blessed in my first 10 years of practice to help a myriad of amazing patients from various musculoskeletal symptoms to extremity issues, to now seeing depression, anxiety, headaches, migraines, vertigo, dizziness, learning issues, and immune-compromised patients, to many more conditions. The personal reward of helping a patient on a healing journey is amazing, and it still inspires me to learn more and keep a smile on my face daily.

What I have come to ultimately realize is that the people are living in a continual state of constant low-level stress, causing a massive unnatural shift in their health. With this realization, functional neurology has become my key to truly unlocking the innate response to balancing the autonomic nervous system in a way that helps stabilize and optimize my patients.

Envision that within you since the moment you graced this world, you harvested a supercomputer responsible for everything you do, think and create. This brain would have the ability to control all of your organs and muscles, create and inspire your thoughts and feelings, and allow you to adapt to any environment. The power of your amazing brain is cosmic, and its rewiring capabilities to adapt and change is fantastic when augmented. Think of a moment that really moved you and was emotional, for instance, the night you met your spouse, the moment your child was born, your first kiss, your first day of college or work. All of these are examples that have hardwired a neurological symphony that encodes a full topographic sequence of events that includes all of the senses. Yet, if asked what was done yesterday or last week, how much detail is recalled? Not much. Why? Herein lies the subtle beauty and complexity of your brain to systematize and organize its neuronal energy in such an innate, amazing way to better serve you.

Imagine if we could start to appreciate this natural pheno-menon as a tool, to better communicate with your body so that improved health, emotion, energy, hormones, affect, metabolic rate and memory, etc. can be achieved. So, now you should start to think about the password to unlock your own greatness from within, and how to facilitate the capabilities of your brain. Can the abilities of your body truly be altered towards health and wellness and move away from symptoms and diseases? The answer is yes; by increasing the probabilities of health from within by magically aligning your spine and thereby maximally firing the quanta of mechanoreceptors of that joint, you innately optimize the upload of messages to the brain, thereby improving the chances of success and rejuvenating health.

Can the secrets of health truly lie from within and completely be controlled by a three-pound brain that contains around 100 billion neurons? Can the health answers we have all been seeking really be contained within a collection of interconnected neurons and conduits? The amazing truth is *yes* and *yes*.

I am happy to inform you that the entire field of science called functional neurology focuses on this. These doctors have learned many ways to use a myriad of functional biometrics to understand the function of your brain, and even more accurately, its constituents. To better understand the complexity of this macrocosmic information, a series of functional tests will be performed on you with the intent to test various parts of your brain, brainstem, balance mechanism, and spinal performance via your spine and nervous system. With the information observed, a functional neurological diagnosis can be assessed to get to the root cause of your symptoms or dysfunction, and then a creation of your optimal care plan can be systematized in accordance to your total health and a happy, healthy brain.

Let's visualize a classic couple in society, where she suffers from headaches, motion sickness, dizziness, intermittent neck pain, and a growing feeling of anxiousness in various life situations that worsens with age. He feels daily low back pain, chronic stomach problems, has high blood pressure, erectile dysfunction, and depression. Does this sound familiar for you or someone you know? What has happened in society that this couple is the new normal? What would be their normal treatment? It would probably be a series of medications from a slew of various medical doctors. Is better physical health and brain health really going to be achieved through better chemistry?

Have any of your friends and family ever been fully treated by a completely different approach? One in which a doctor of the future can truly oversee the case though completion and watch a patient be nurtured on their own wellness journey?

This is what I am blessed to do daily. My classical training as a chiropractor set the stage to understand the spine and nervous system. This further led me on a journey to work with high-level athletes by understanding the subtle truth of the peripheral nervous system and extremities. Next, I studied the caring and nurturing of pregnancy and delicate pediatric patients. My voyage continued with the study of functional neurology, vestibular rehabilitation, and mastering the migraine. These studies have been my own path to better help and understand patients over the last 17 years.

In reference to the previous example of the couple, this is truly treatable and even fun under the right care. The way I view this in my practice would be to create a feeling of wonder and magic while wielding science and logic to unlock the quintessential elegance of the nervous system, by taking patients on a journey from the known to the unknown and then back to the known of the body and brain. This method increases the probability of finding the true cause of the symptoms, as stated previously.

As the brain starts to repair and remodel, a beautiful thing starts to happen. Biometrics start to strengthen, symptoms start to reduce, and the body starts to feel improved and invigorated. Bodily movements start to become fluidlike again, and patients start to increase their ability to handle daily stressors, mood and global affect improve, and the whole body becomes more efficient. Sounds fascinating, right? Who would have thought that a body that works more optimally by improved communication to the brain can respond so beautifully? Sages, shamans, and copious healers have stated this for many decades, even centuries. So how is it that we have slipped too far down the path towards an unhealthy brain? Our culture always moves faster and faster, and at a quickened rate, while food became easier and unhealthy. Technology keeps growing, but at what expense to our brain health from electromagnetic frequency pattern interruptions and water contamination from increased pollution? What about increased, daily job stress to keep up with our neighbors and many further bodily stressors such as drugs, medications, vapes, genetically modified food and more obesity than ever recorded on our planet? Now that you're thinking *wow, that sounds grim and depressing*, here is the great news: it is mostly all preventable and treatable. So whatever level of your current health and lifestyle you have been enjoying or trapped in, now is the time to make a change. Now is the perfect time to recreate your healthy brain!

The first steps will appear easy, but it will actually be extremely hard for most of you because of the current way you have hardwired your brain. The first step is your decision to change, with the second step creating an action plan to move towards health and a new life. Neural pruning is the next step through a sequence of repetitive, positive processes to create new neuronal pathways of wellness, and pruning your old, common, sickly ones. This is how you can really start to make change to a new you. When you compound that with my five pillars of health I have pragmatically seen, miracles are truly yours for the taking.

The five pillars that I write about at length in my last book, *Functional Living*, are as follows:

Pillar One: A properly working nervous system
Pillar Two: Proper exercise
Pillar Three: Proper nutrition
Pillar Four: A proper mental attitude
Pillar Five: Proper rest and relaxation

These five pillars encapsulate your wellness blueprint to feeling physiologically younger than your chronological age. Envision your life for a moment as one in which you wake up most days and feel great and ready to take on your day, instead of the day taking you on. It can all start with your decision to act and finding a wellness captain to help you motivate and navigate you on your wellness cruise.

Each day we all interact with people that are sadly struggling with many symptoms that hold them back and do not allow them to perform and live optimally. My dream is that I can inspire and educate you to move towards this new healthy reality by setting the scene of what is possible. By understanding the inner workings of your brain and body and being present and taking responsibility for your own health, you are unstoppable. You are more equipped than you know, and by getting your brain and nervous system checked, you can find out possible pitfalls before they happen. This concept of optimizing your brain and its connections to your body is not futuristic; it is currently present right now. I have been chosen and am honored to be able to understand this material to make it fun and exciting to my current and future patients. The truth of the way our brains function is fascinating and amazing, and when examined and corrected the right way, it appears to be like modern day wizardry. Let's all aspire to create a future generation that is healthier than we are. To do that, we have to take drastic, positive steps in our culture. This can start right now! Once you feel the difference of your brain starting to feel healthier, the empowering nature will be contagious. Let's start the ride of positive functioning neuronal connections that all interact and communicate the way they were designed to. From the first order neuronal message all the way down the hierarchy of the second and third, it eventually connects with its end target, and then innately stamping its message ticket for the return trip. This incredible, proper nervous system communication is the key to internal prosperity, proper organ function, a properly functioning musculoskeletal system, and a globally faster, more effective healing human. This will allow us as a society to possibly become free of daily medications as a first resort and using the five pillars of health as our daily medicine instead.

The power of the brain is cosmic, and unleashing its potential is our true destiny. Always remember that every brilliantly designed brain program was created for a purpose, and that purpose when used correctly can restore our population as a whole back to wellness and a collection of happy brains swimming in a sea of happiness.

It has been an honor to share my thoughts with you, and

I hope that you take them as a stimulus to move forward and start to really enjoy life. If you are interested in learning more about my work, please visit my website at www.leonchiropractic. com and follow us on all social media platforms for cutting-edge health information.

Yours in Health,

Jared A. Leon, D.C., C.C.E.P., F.I.C.P.A, F.A.B.V.R. and Board Eligible Functional Neurology Diplomat

About the Author

Dr. Jared A Leon

Dr. Leon has embraced his work with a passion rarely seen in the healthcare community. Rather than focusing on a patient's particular symptoms, Dr. Leon concentrates upon the innate wellness harbored within the human body, thus allowing the body's natural and powerful forces to overcome afflictions.

He performs his work non-invasively, with gentle external corrections of one's own architecture to restore neural pathways from interference. Since it is ultimately these pathways that govern our health and well-being, he reinforces and facilitates the neurological system's natural ability to maintain a body's health.

Dr. Leon firmly believes it is the duty of a healthcare professional to maintain wellness, by rooting out the cause of health problems, not just treating the symptoms of an illness. He strives to restore the body to peak performance, thereby minimizing the chance of illness and its debilitating results.

Contact Information:
Leon Chiropractic
213 Hallock Rd.
Suite 4B
Stony Brook, NY 11790
631-689-1000
www.leonchiropractic.com
drjared5@gmail.com

ATTITUDE & ENERGY!!!

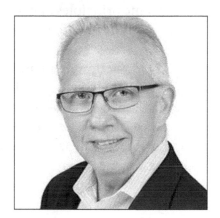

Dr. Gerald J Agasar

Over the years, I have been described as a "little guy with a lot of energy." I grew up in North Philly in a family of five children. There was always a lot of activity, and as a child, I learned that I needed to work hard for the things I wanted in my life because no one was going to hand me success.

As a young man, I used to apologize for my intensity during my formative years. When people would talk about my intensity, it made me feel as though it was a bad thing. I now realize that I was not as comfortable with myself as I could or should have been, which is why I took those comments personally. But it was that very energy that led to many successes in academics and sports. According to my SAT scores, I had average intelligence, but I worked very hard in school, which paid off as I was ranked in the top 10% of my high school class. I was an avid sports guy, but not being blessed with God-given talent or size (being 5'5" and 140 pounds in high school), I had to work hard to be a starter on the football team my senior year. As a defensive back, I performed well and was part of the team, even though I was not the 5'10", 173-pound player the program listed me as. We still laugh about that embellishment 45 years later!

After attending two years at Ursinus College, a small liberal arts college in Pennsylvania where I was studying pre-med, I decided to attend National College of Chiropractic and, following in my father's footsteps, completed my schooling to become a chiropractor. I used the same principles of hard work and intense energy as I had to this point in my life to achieve high levels of success.

As I came out of chiropractic school and began my career, my work ethic and energy along with my passion for chiropractic helped me to build a practice where I was serving my community as well as surrounding areas in a very positive way. I am actually the longest-tenured chiropractor in my chosen town and have now been in continuous practice there for more than 37 years. In those early years, it was definitely my attitude and energy that helped me build a successful practice. I was confident enough to believe that success would continue indefinitely.

I enjoy sports and competition, and I use a lot of sports analogies in my practice, but I never seemed to be prepared for the curveballs of life. We all have them, some bigger than others. While we may have similar situations, we all experience these curveballs in different ways. Yet it is how we respond to them that determines the direction of our future. Will we be positive or negative?

Energy can be both positive and negative. There are scores of books that have been written and hundreds of inspirational speakers who claim to teach the difference between positive and negative energy. Positivity breeds positivity while negativity breeds negativity. It is a simple concept when you think about it, but one that is hard to wrap your head around when you are in the midst of a challenge, that curveball I am referring to.

I will admit that my energy was not always positive. In fact, I can say without a doubt that there were times in my life that I was a hothead and a sore loser. In those early years, I did not handle life's curveballs with grace and positivity. In fact, when I had a failed relationship that I did not anticipate, I grew despondent. My life was sailing along a fantastic trajectory, and all of a sudden, BOOM, I found myself a failure. Okay, failure is a bit strong, but I was young and pretty low from the experience and the crushing emotional blow I felt. I found myself in a bad place; no one could help me out of it but me, and I had no idea how to do that. It was a time when my energy was low, and I was in emotional pain. Have you ever been in emotional hell with no light showing you the way out? It's not a fun place to be, but my guess is every person puts themselves in just such a place at some point in their life, maybe even more than once. I know that no emotional or physical pain is ever exactly the same, but we can certainly empathize with one another when we experience it.

Somehow, through the depths of my pain, I knew I did not want to stay there. There had to be a better way. I wish I could tell you how I found the most profound book I ever read. It was truly a turning point for me in learning how powerful attitude and energy really could be in my life. The book *The Power of Positive Thinking* by Norman Vincent Peale absolutely **woke me up!** (In my humble opinion, it should absolutely be required reading for every high school student in America.) I read it over and over and over again. I had read other books on positive thinking and how to create a positive mindset, but this one really impacted me. It made me rethink how I approach life and pointed me in a direction that would bring new purpose to my life and my practice.

As I said, I did <u>not</u> like feeling down, so not only reading this book but connecting with its principles brought new meaning to the way I was living. As I started to apply the principles to my daily life, my moods improved, my outlook became more positive, and I found reasons to be thankful. I certainly did not come out of that dark place over night, but by applying those tried and true principles every day, I did come back with an attitude and energy that I thought would carry me through a lifetime. There is a direct correlation to happy thoughts and positive outcomes, and I was in control of those thoughts.

As I came out of that dark place, I was blessed with a chiropractic practice in the top 15% of my profession. I loved serving my patients every day and enjoyed being a fixture in my community. But most of all, I loved being a father to my three children and raising them to be polite, positive, and productive individuals. Notice that I did not say perfect. As I had learned and applied a positive attitude to all aspects of my life, I thought it was only fitting to incorporate the same concepts into my parenting as well. I encouraged each of my children to do their best, like most parents do, but also encouraged them to find positivity and gratitude all around them. Don't get me wrong, I wanted to see my children succeed and get good grades, but it was not the A's on the report card that excited me as much as the teacher's comments such as, "Displays a positive attitude!" I knew that would be more beneficial to their success in life than just getting good grades.

Yes, I thought I had life figured out. I understood my calling. I was passionate about getting people on the road to wellness. I had a wonderful family and had committed my life to Christ. I did not think life could get much better: a pretty wife, beautiful and healthy kids, great practice getting lots of people well, money in the bank, and just six payments left on my house. That is when life threw me a huge curveball, one that I tried to avoid, but could not.

On the outside, my marriage looked great, but on the inside, I knew it was not healthy. As my world crumbled before my eyes, I realized the only things I could control were my attitude and energy, the things I knew connected me to my calling and my lifestyle. Although I had faced challenges before, this one felt bigger than all the others put together. Painful does not begin to describe how I felt, and it nearly destroyed me not to see my children 50 percent of the time. The crossroads of this curveball brought me to a choice: become angry and bitter toward the mother of my children, an attitude that would ultimately destroy me, or rise above, find the positive, and continue forward. I had three sets of eyes watching me, looking to me for reassurance that life would somehow be all right. The choice was clear.

There were days in the early years following the separation and divorce that I would put them on the bus, walk back to the house, and fall into a black hole of sadness. Initially I thought of what I had lost and felt horrible; this practice did not serve me well. I was miserable. I was like a zombie. My vibration was very low, and I was just existing. It wasn't a good feeling. I wasn't helping anyone. I got tired of feeling that way and through my faith in Jesus and with the help of people that loved and supported me, I finally chose a different mindset. I eventually chose to be healthy, joyful, and not be sad. I pivoted my attitude to think about all that I was (and am) grateful for: my life, my health, my three beautiful gifts from God that are my children, and my ability to make a good living serving others. The more I focused on what I had rather than what I had lost, the more alive I felt, and that carried me through.

Although the divorce was difficult in so many ways, I did not want to become jaded towards the opposite sex. My faith in Jesus Christ tells me that I am to love others the way I love myself and to put my trust in Him. It was not an easy decision because I was still the "little guy with a lot of energy," but I liked the way I felt when my mind and body worked together to maintain a positive mental attitude and energy in my daily living and the way I served my patients and community.

As a chiropractor, I work with people to remove interferences to their nervous system so their bodies can function more efficiently and optimally. Early in my career, I learned that even if I gave the best spinal adjustment to each person I saw, they would not get the best results if they were in an unhealthy emotional state; their recovery process would get stuck. Today, there is a ton of research showing the benefits of positive thinking and its relationship to improving healthy outcomes—not only with neck and back pain, but with more significant health conditions like cancer.

After more than 30 years and now being a three-generation chiropractic family as my eldest son has joined me in practice, we educate our patients on the importance of brain balance as part of the healing process to achieve the best results. Negative thoughts and emotions put us in sympathetic tone (survival mode), while positive thoughts and emotions put us in a more parasympathetic tone (healing mode). It is the simple, happy, positive thoughts that allow for better patient outcomes.

Learning how to care for the body so it can function optimally has been my passion for my entire career. It is the connection between mind and body that elevates one's vitality. Even though there were times in my first 50 years I did not consciously think about that connection, I now know it was at the core of my being. It is all about waking up and realizing that the connection between the brain and the spine is real; the connection between the spine and positive emotions is powerful, and my life—my health—is best served when I keep those connections fluid and part of my lifestyle, not just something I pull off the shelf now and again.

Remember that we will all experience challenges in life, some more than others. It will not always be easy, but in more than 37 years of practicing chiropractic and serving thousands and thousands of patients, I know for sure that the attitude and energy you put into your health, your relationships, and your life will greatly affect your outcomes. I belong to a mastermind group with six other awesome chiropractors. We've been meeting for over 16 years, and the last line of our mission statement says, "We realize positive ENERGY, ENERGY, ENERGY will give us momentum for the positive change."

I love it! I live it!!

Every day, I *choose* to be positive and energetic. After 12 years of single parenthood, I have been blessed to meet and marry the partner of my dreams. We share the same values, a strong faith, and positivity. We laugh and love together as we handle this journey called life. She has a great attitude and energy! We are the proud parents of six children, and we have just opened a new holistic wellcare practice together called Agasar Family WellCare at Inner Spa, and we are very excited for the future!

You—only you—control your attitude and energy! Stay positive. The world will try to bring you down, but trust in being positive. Stay with it. The Universe will reward you! I am living proof that no matter what life throws at you, when you listen to your gut, when you lean on the spirit above, and when you stay positive and do not let the negativity of the world seep into your thinking, your future is bright and full of vibrancy! It just may take a little longer than you hoped. Stay the course!

Never, ever give up. You never know when the BEST part of your life is just around the next bend.

About the Author

Dr. Gerald J Agasar

Dr. Jerry is a second-generation chiropractor who has been practicing in Newtown, Pennsylvania, for over 37 years. His passion is serving and educating his community on living the chiropractic healthy lifestyle, teaching the importance of good posture as well as good alignment, and mobility of the spine to maximize the function of your nervous system. Doing this in conjunction with good nutrition, moderate exercise, and maintaining a positive outlook will greatly improve your health outcomes!

He lives a very active lifestyle, and enjoys biking, skiing and tennis. He enjoys having a positive impact on children, either in the classroom or on the athletic field. He has been very active in Rotary since 1983, modeling their mission "service above self," and along with his fellow Rotarians has collected over 2,500 used bicycles to be donated to third-world countries. He and his wife, Cathy, share a common purpose in helping others become a better version of themselves every day.

Contact Information:
Agasar Family WellCare at Inner Spa
The Atrium
4 Terry Dr. Ste. 13
Newtown, PA 18940
Website: agasarfamilywellcare.com
Telephone: (215) 550-6502

SAVING YOUR BRAIN

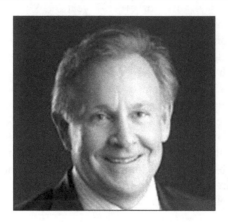

Dr. Kelly Miller

When I graduated from Logan University of Health Sciences in 1980, it was generally accepted that we were born with so many neurons (brain cells) and we just whittled away at them as we aged based on our traumas, toxins, and thoughts. We now know that this is not true. In fact, we retain the ability to regenerate our neurons throughout our lifetime. This process is called neurogenesis. This single fact should bring hope to everyone, especially those who have been diagnosed with or those caretakers for those diagnosed with ADHD, Autism Spectrum Disorder, PTSD (Post Traumatic Stress Disorder), TBI (Traumatic Brain Injury), anxiousness, depression, and cognitive decline from Alzheimer's and Parkinson's. The question we should be asking ourselves is, "How can I enhance neurogenesis in my own brain?"

I began noticing some significant cognitive decline in my mid-fifties. I had always loved watching old movies. I could remember all the names of the actors and actresses and the plot of each movie. I had always been able to keep a clock and calendar in my head. I have traveled to many countries and visited many cities. Gradually, I experienced more difficulty putting names to faces of the people in the movies, forgetting important dates, and an inability to recall the name of the city when looking at the many pictures taken when I was there. I even found myself driving past exits if I was talking to someone on the phone. Other things were happened. I became more serious, critical, impatient, and would have episodes of anger. I used to be more happy-go-lucky.

What was going on? These alarming changes in my memory and mood initiated my personal search to save my own brain. My earlier years of excess drug and alcohol abuse in the 60s and 70s and playing rugby for 20 years had taken their toll. I calculate that over the span of 20 years, I was involved in close to 10,000 tackles. I began researching and reading every natural remedy therapy for improving cognitive function because 350 drug trials had offered no solution for arresting Alzheimer's. In 2015, I had my first brain mapping. I was having trouble hearing and the doctor asked me how many concussions I had in the past. He told me that the part of my brain that processed hearing had been damaged and was not working well. After working on my brain with an audio-visual and treatment device called BrainTap for 60 days, I was no longer having the delayed hearing effect. It is interesting to note that I have been told by many patients who wore hearing aids that their hearing improved more after we used the BrainTap on their brains than after they got their hearing aids.

After three years of research I published my fourth book, *Saving your Brain: Causes, Prevention, and Reversal of Dementia/ Alzheimer's* in August 2018. During these three years of research, I visited many brain-based clinics to gain more knowledge. I evaluated the efficacy of all the technologies in the book on my patients using heart rate variability and a functional cardiovascular assessment device called Max Pulse for two years. My criteria for accepting a protocol was that whatever we did for the patient must improve their circulation and the function of the healing part of the nervous system called the parasympathetic nervous system (rest and digest).

Heart rate variability is a measurement of the vital signs of your nervous system. The nervous system is divided into three parts: the emergency or survival part called the sympathetic, the healing part or rest and digest part called the parasympathetic, and the central nervous system/neuro-hormonal part. I tell my patients that this test will show them how well they are handling stress or how stress is handling them. Unfortunately, for 90 % of us, it is the latter. Yes, nine out of ten patients we scan with HRV are locked into survival (fight/flight) physiology. No wonder there are so many people suffering from anxiousness, digestive issues, and sleep problems. Survival physiology produces adrenaline and cortisol. The prolonged production of cortisol kills neurons.

The Max Pulse is an instrument that measures four different aspects of cardiovascular function. These functions are rated on a percentile compared to other people of the same sex and age in North America. One of the four parts assessed is something called arterial elasticity. Arterial elasticity measures the ability of the blood vessel to expand (dilate). Loss of this function is a predictor of future cardiovascular events such as heart attacks and strokes. The brain uses 25% of the cardiac output, 20% of the oxygen, and 25% of the glucose produced in our bodies. Optimum blood flow is vital to supply your brain with oxygen, fuel in the form of glucose and fatty acids, and micronutrients to supply the raw materials for mitochondrial energy needs and for the brain tissue. Mitochondria are the power plant within the cells; they produce all the energy that each cell needs.

Every recommendation made for our patients had to be effective 80% or more of the time in improving circulation and the power of the healing part of the nervous system or it was abandoned.

In the title, S-A-V-I-N-G Y-O-U-R B-R-A-I-N, each letter is an acronym for something important and necessary for optimum brain function. Each acronym can be a negative or positive risk factor depending on how you are doing in that category. To change the brain for the better, you need to improve each area of deficiency until there is a tipping point that enhances neurogenesis.

S is for sleep. Proper sleep is critical for optimum brain function in maintaining or restoring cognitive function. There are five stages of sleep that are cycled through each night. Each stage should accumulate about 90 minutes throughout a sleep cycle. The delta stage is critical for metabolically cleaning the brain via the brain's lymph system. Think about a sponge lying on the bottom of your kitchen sink picking up the debris from the plates, pots, and pans you rinse before putting them in the dishwasher. You need to put soap and fresh water on the sponge and squeeze it to clean it. This is similar to the process that delta sleep does for your brain. It gets rid of all the waste material from the cells. If you consistently sleep less than six hours or more than nine hours, research demonstrates you are increasing cognitive decline and decreasing your longevity. The optimum sweet spot for most people seems to be 7.6 hours of sleep.

Is a lack of sleep causing the brain problem or is the brain problem causing the disruption of sleep? This a big debate in science right now. It is similar to the question of, "Which came first the chicken or the egg?" I am of the belief that insomnia is a reflection or indication of an underlying brain problem. The reason I say this is that when we set out to correct a brain imbalance with neurofeedback, audio-visual entrainment, nutrition, and sleep improve. Getting proper sleep is critical to optimum brain and neuron nervous system function. Our peak healing times are from 10:00 p.m. to 2:00 a.m. This is when the parasympathetic (rest and digest) nervous system is most active. This is when we produce substances like melatonin (the most powerful antioxidant in the body) and growth hormone. When we don't sleep during these times, our brain health suffers.

I put a great emphasis on correcting sleep patterns. I encourage my patients to go to bed at sundown and rise with the sun as much as possible. This also helps restore normal circadian rhythms of all the hormones in the body.

A is for Autonomic balance or imbalance for most of us. The autonomic (or automatic) part of our nervous system is made up of the sympathetic nervous and parasympathetic nervous systems. It regulates all our organ functions automatically. In an emergency, the survival nervous system activates adrenaline, followed by cortisol. Adrenaline first activates fatty acids from fat stores for energy expenditure and secondarily with cortisol to produce more glucose. This is supposed to be for short-term duration; this may be from seconds, to minutes, to maybe a few hours. Unfortunately, we find that 90% of Americans are staying in survival physiology most of the time when they are assessed with heart rate variability. The bottom line is that constant cortisol production kills neurons. We use heart rate variability to monitor progress in achieving a shift to the healing part of the nervous system. There are multiple therapies that will help achieve this shift: breathing in for three to four seconds followed by exhaling six to eight seconds, gargling, oxytocin, P.E.M.F. (pulsed electromagnetic frequency), and the hummingbird exercise. Helping the nervous system to increase the parasympathetic part of the nervous system helps the brain function better.

V is for vitamins, minerals, and antioxidants. You need to be eating organic vegetables, fruits, and meats. Avoid GMO (genetically modified) foods, packaged foods containing aspartame, MSG (monosodium glutamate), and trans-fats. Around 1950, the average orange contained 50mg of Vitamin C. Today, an orange contains about 5mg of Vitamin C. This is because we have depleted the mineral content in the soil because we never let it rest between harvests. We need supplementation in today's world. Besides Vitamins A, B, C, D, and E, our bodies require minerals like magnesium, zinc, selenium, manganese, and antioxidants like curcumin, ginseng, resveratrol, and others. Adequate fatty acids, particularly DHA, can reduce the risk of Alzheimer's by as much as 49%. I have never tested a patient yet that had adequate fatty acids.

I is for Inflammation/infection. You need to evaluate blood markers for C-reactive protein and homocysteine. Elevations of these markers is bad for the brain. Elevated homocysteine indicates a deficiency in B vitamins. This can be caused by genetic variants like MTFHR and/or deficiency in the diet. Supplementation of Methylated B Vitamins is important for most people. C-reactive protein can be reduced with Omega 3 high in DHA, curcumin, and resveratrol. More importantly, you need to find what is causing the inflammation/infection. Food/chemical allergies/sensitivities are a common cause as well as environmental toxins like mercury, aluminum, glyphosates

(Roundup), herbicides, pesticides, plastics from contaminated air, and water sources. When you get a CBC (complete blood cell count) check the percentages of monocytes and eosinophils. If the monocytes are over 7%, you have a chronic infection somewhere. If your eosinophils are over 3%, you have a chronic allergy.

Mold infections are common. One in four people have a gene variant that does not readily recognize mold in the body and a problem with mounting an adequate immune response. Mold infections are commonly found in the sinuses, lungs, and GI tract. There is a visual acuity test on www.survivingmold.com that can detect mold infections with a high percentage of accuracy. If you fail this test, seek help with a provider that is knowledgeable on helping you to get rid of mold infections. The presence of mold in the body gives rises to many bacterial infections.

N is for your neuro hormones. Your hormones influence the neurotransmitters in your brain. Adequate testosterone in men and estrogen in women is critical for the production of dopamine, which is found in large amounts in the frontal cortex or the executive decision- making part of your brain. Alzheimer's patients have low dopamine levels. Low thyroid levels are common in the aging population. Routine blood work alone is not adequate to diagnose low thyroid function. Check your basal body temperature in the early morning for three to five mornings. If it is consistently less than 98.2 degrees, chances are good you have hypo-thyroid function. Better yet, find a provider who uses the Thyroflex device. The Thyroflex is an FDA-cleared instrument that measures intracellular, bioactive T3 levels in nerve and muscle cells through the brachioradialis reflex. This test is considered 98.5% accurate. Healthy thyroid function reduces Alzheimer's risk by 50%.

G is for genetic variants. If you have a family history of Alzheimer's, you should get genetic testing. The most common genetic variant involved with Alzheimer's is the APOE4 gene variant. Approximately 50% of Alzheimer's patients have this gene variant. APOE is an LDL that is responsible for binding to Abeta and taking it from the brain to the liver to be processed through the bile and through the stool. The APOE4 gene variant is less efficient in doing this when compared to the APOE2 or the APOE3 gene variants. No worries, the APOE4 gene variant is actionable. If you take niacin, exercise regularly, and keep your fasting glucose levels below 95, you can compensate for the APOE4 gene variant.

Y is for your belief system. What you think is probably the most important factor in your brain health. When we look at the bottom 10% of individuals on a stress scale compared to the top 10%, there is a 400% increased risk factor for cognitive decline and Alzheimer's in the higher-level stress group. Your adaptability to destress is critical to your brain health. You must learn to replace your fears with faith. Stay in the present time. Forgive the past and be hopeful of the future. I tell patients I cannot keep them from the stress they are having, but we can help keep stress from damaging their brains and nervous systems.

O is for obesity and oxidative stress. The bottom line is the more fat in our bodies, the more the inflammation we have and the smaller the brain becomes. Seek help to shed a few extra pounds and keep them off by adapting new eating patterns and adopting stress reduction techniques.

U is for unfriendly environment. This is an area that is almost universally under-addressed by both doctors and patients. There are about 10,000 chemicals in our environment that did not exist before World War II. The toxins are in the air you breathe, the food you eat, and the water you drink. This can be greatly reduced by adequate water and air filtration systems. See www.drkellymiller.com/9-variables-of-health and click on "What You Drink" and "What You Breathe" for more information.

R is for reading. Research demonstrates that reading helps preserve cognitive function.

B is for blood flow. In over 15,000 SPECT images of the brain, Dr. Daniel Amen has conclusively proven that chronic brain problems and cognitive decline exhibit dramatic changes in the circulation in the brain. All of our patients are scanned by a device called the Max Pulse to determine their cardiovascular capabilities. Improving circulation is essential to help carry oxygen, micronutrients, and fuel in the form of glucose or fatty acids that the brain needs. Optimizing cardiovascular function is critical to maintain cognitive function or restoring loss of function. Multiple strategies are used to improve the integrity of blood vessels, cardiac output, and arterial elasticity. Good blood flow to the brain is vital.

R is for repetitive head injury. If you have been involved in contact sports or car crashes, it is imperative you get assessed immediately and develop preventative, restorative strategies for nutritional support and circulation restoration of your brain. A single concussion can double your risk for Alzheimer's. A loss of consciousness couple with the APOE 4 gene increases your risk tenfold for Alzheimer's. These injuries can be compensated for with the proper administration of the multiple technologies now available.

A is for activity or exercise. The research is overwhelming, indicating that exercise helps preserve cognitive function. Find an exercise you like and do it regularly. Variety is the spice of life; alternating your exercise routine and challenging yourself to do new activities improves your brain function.

I is for insulin resistance/sensitivity. Half of all Alzheimer's patients demonstrate blood sugar dysregulation. Alzheimer's has been called Type III diabetes by some. Keeping your fasting blood glucose levels below 95 will go a long way in keeping your brain healthy. Work with a healthcare provider that will help you achieve this. Diet, exercise, supplementation, and stress management with an audio-visual trainer are all helpful. Blood sugar regulation is a key to preserving or restoring cognitive function and preventing Alzheimer's.

N is for neurotransmitters. When we conduct brain mapping, we measure five different brain waves: delta, theta, alpha, low beta, and high beta. These brain waves are reflective of the neurotransmitters. For example, excessive levels of dopamine can cause high alpha and beta waves. When brain waves are abnormal, the neurotransmitters are imbalanced. These imbalances are often manifested in symptoms of anxiousness, attention deficit, or depression. These symptoms are increased risk factors for cognitive decline in Alzheimer's. In the vast majority of cases (almost everyone), these brain imbalances can be corrected by non-drug therapies such as core strengthening, balance therapy, neurofeedback, audiovisual treatment, infrared light therapy, chiropractic adjustments, acupuncture, and nutritional and/or hormonal therapies.

Prevention is always the best and optimum action for preventing cognitive decline in Alzheimer's and keeping a happy brain. However, the brain is resilient and neuroplastic. Your brain can change with the correct thoughts and activities. If you make positive changes in the areas of deficiency and weakness and use light and sound therapy, your brain can change, even late in life!

About the Author

Dr. Kelly Miller

Dr. Miller is a chiropractic physician, as well as a naturopathic physician. He also holds certifications in acupuncture and functional medicine and a fellowship in aging and regenerative medicine.

Contact Information:
Websites: www.drkellymiller.com, www.savingyourbrain.com

Clinics in Kansas City, Missouri, Tampa and Naples, Florida

BEYOND WHAT WAS: ACHIEVING RESILIENCE AND A HAPPY BRAIN

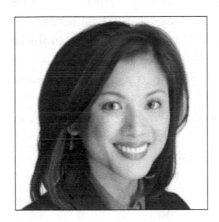

Dr. Kim Hoang

Growing up, I didn't have many material objects, but I had my family. My parents were immigrants, fleeing South Vietnam during the Fall of Saigon in 1975. My two oldest siblings, my brother and sister, were five and two. My mom was pregnant with my brother, Alex. They fled on a boat filled with many other immigrants. They weren't sure where they were going or if they would be able to eat again. Many days at sea, they were simply trying to survive. I didn't get a chance to know all of the details because my parents didn't talk about it much when I was growing up. I am not sure if it is because they wanted to block it out or if they didn't think it was important to share at the time.

I was born in New Orleans and I am the fifth of seven children. We lived in an area called East New Orleans, or as the Vietnamese would say, "Viet Sai" or Versailles. I don't remember much living there because I was five years old when we moved down to the bayou in a small Louisiana town called Houma. There, I went to elementary school and eventually high school.

The population of Houma at the time was about 30,000. Growing up in a very small town was difficult at times. There weren't many Vietnamese (or Asians for that matter). During my junior high school years of seventh and eighth grade, some of the kids were very ruthless. They would say things like "Ching chong" and I wasn't respected. I didn't have much self-confidence and I would go home and cry to my mother.

My parents worked very hard manual jobs to supply a roof over our heads and food on the table. My dad had many odd end jobs ranging from shrimping and crabbing to painting the oil rigs. He would be out at sea, sometimes working for a couple weeks before he was able to make it back home to see the family for a couple days, before going back out to sea again. My mom shucked oysters for a living. At times they would work between 10 and 14 hours a day.

My parents really tried their best to give us a good life. Unfortunately, with bad investments in a shrimping boat that sank and having no insurance, we always lived in debt. My parents passed away young; my mom was 48 and my dad at 51. I was 21 at the time when my mom passed. At that time, I was in my second of nine trimesters at Parker Chiropractic in Dallas, Texas. I felt helpless for my mom.

When she was dying in the hospital, I didn't know much about why her health was failing as I had just started chiropractic school. I am still uncertain as to how and why she actually died and didn't know much medically, because my dad didn't want to do autopsy. When I was growing up, she was very fragile. One day she would be fine and next day she would be shivering in bed. I believe she always had a weak immune system. From what I understand, she contracted Legionnaires' disease, a bacterial infection sometimes spread through air conditioning ducts and sprinklers in the produce section of grocery stores. Usually a healthy person would be able to fight it off, but she was unable to and her body started to shut down.

My dad was the same age as my mom. He was your typical Vietnamese man and didn't show much emotion. However, when my mom passed, there was that emotional side of him that poured out to his seven children. He usually never calls any of his kids, but after mom's death, he played the role of Mr. Mom. He began to call us just to check up on us. After mom's death, four out of us seven siblings didn't live at home anymore.

My siblings and I encouraged him to get a physical checkup just so we could have him with us for a longer time. Although he was more emotional with us, he was still the typical Vietnamese "stubborn" man. He was very religious and said, "When God calls me, it is time to go." He was a heavy smoker. Three years later, he had a thrombotic stoke that left him paralyzed on the right side of his body. He needed a feeding tube and had a tracheotomy placed because he needed help with breathing. He couldn't talk to us, so we used alphabet board to help us communicate with him. I am currently 42 at the time of writing this and my experience with my parents has been one half of my life. My experience growing up taught me to put school first, have financial security, and live a healthy life.

I was in two motor vehicle collisions at the ages of 8 and 13. I never went to a doctor because I was young, and my parents didn't know to take me to one. Since I was one of seven kids, we didn't have transportation or have time to see the doctor. I remembered in middle school, I complained of having low back pain to my mom. My mother told me I was growing old fast and just to deal with it. I would just take over the counter NSAIDS like Advil and BC powder. It didn't help much.

My first year of college was at Louisiana State University ... I wasn't sure what to major in. I knew I wanted to be a doctor, but I wasn't sure what specialty I wanted to pursue. I then went to see Dr. Celine, a chiropractor, and asked her questions about the field. I became her patient and she also became my mentor. Dr. Celine is about five feet tall and she is full of energy. After a couple of weeks of treatment, my lower back felt so much better. I then started to work out and watched what I ate. I was excited to be pain-free through natural and conservative care. After my experience with Dr. Celine, I knew I wanted to be a chiropractor. After graduating from chiropractic school, I was an associate for a chiropractor for about four years when I decided it was time for me to open up my own office. I was scared because I didn't have much business experience. After a couple of years in private practice, I was able to open my second office. After many years of hard work, I was able to achieve financial freedom.

Currently, I live in the New Orleans, Louisiana area. Let's face it, we aren't the healthiest population on the planet. However, I try to live a healthy life. We see many patients that range from low back, neck, disc herniations, headache, and extremity pain. I have a team of three doctors, and we incorporate the decompression table, which helps with disc and facet issues, dry needling, which helps with trigger points, BrainTap, and massage therapy.

This book is about how to have a healthy brain. Recently I purchased and use what is called BrainTap. It is a state-of-the-art light therapy. It can help with many issues that range from weight loss to addictions. I personally use it for meditation.

In the last five years, I went through a divorce and a tough relationship after the divorce. I didn't really know what anxiety was before these life experiences. The BrainTap has helped me meditate. I also believe in working out to maintain not just optimal physical health but mental health. When I have a stressful day, I would go to the gym to decompress. I believe in getting regular adjustments of the spine, massage therapy, dry needling, BrainTap, and working out. I do love to eat but feel that you can experience new food without getting off track. I choose vegetable dishes and avoid fried or creamy food. I like to eat in small quantities and eat often, sometimes five times per day. Anyone that knows me, knows I always have a little stash of food, so I don't get hungry and overeat.

My siblings have been my rock. I have five other siblings (two brothers and three sisters) and about 15 nieces and nephews. We remain very close. Upon my father's death, he wanted for us to promise him that we would always stay together as a family. We try our best to see one another often. It is therapeutic for me to spend time with them. I have no children, but I love to see my nieces and nephews grow up.

I personally believe traveling is important as it allows for me to learn about different cultures and it feeds my soul and brain. I didn't travel much as a kid because we didn't have the financial means to do so. So as an adult, I travel as often as I can. Traveling not only helps me decompress, but it also allows for me to learn about different cultures and how others in this world live. Often it gives me a sense of appreciation of how lucky I am to live in the United States of America. I am grateful for the journey my parents took to get us here. I appreciate the opportunity I've been given to live the life I live.

I try to surround myself with positive people and positive energy because it is contagious. In this past year, it has been a healing time for me. I think meditation, acceptance, and forgiveness has helped me get to the place I am today. I believe having a balanced lifestyle is important for a healthy brain. Our brain is the most important organ in our body, so take care of it and it will take care of you. Do so by taking care of yourself physically and mentally.

In closing, I hope my story inspires you to do what you think is unattainable. I didn't grow up with a lot of money. I knew I wanted financial freedom, and I did it through hard work and dedication in school. I wanted to live a healthy life. And being a chiropractor has opened up my world to living the best me!

About the Author

Dr. Kim Hoang

Dr. Hoang is the founder of Hoang Chiropractic Center, with two locations in Metairie and Gretna, Louisiana.

Contact Information:
Email: drhoang@hoangchiro.com
Website: www.hoangchiro.com

THE PURSUIT OF HAPPINESS
HAPPY MIND, HAPPY LIFE

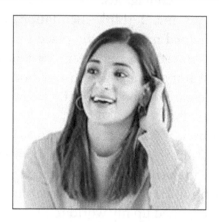

Dr. Lalitaa Suglani

"Happiness does not depend on what we have. It does depend on how we feel towards what we have. We can be happy with little and miserable with much. It is a choice."
-Dr. Lalitaa

Each of us holds unimaginable power within oneself, a power that is so strong, so extraordinary, and so beautiful, which if you tap into and unleash, it can transform you and your overall happiness.

Hey, it is Dr. Lalitaa Suglani here. I work as a psychologist and coach. I support people with their mental health and well-being. I currently live in the UK and frequently travel globally, presenting at seminars and workshops to assist people in discovering and connecting with learning the 'how to' in loving who they are. We are all unique and what creates happiness for one will be different for another. I want you to live life to its fullest and to be happy! I believe we all deserve to be happy and it is often us that stand in our own way. How? Through our core beliefs and values that have been developed from a young age. My main focus is to work with you on understanding and developing your mindset, relationships, health, and wealth to reach your version of success. I love what I do!

Most people whom I work with appear to be holding the question: "How do I become happy?" or, "Where can I find happiness?" Some part of what I do is dedicated to helping people identify what happiness means to them and how to connect with it. Happiness is not a distant bird somewhere in a bush. It is often perching right upon our own shoulder and we often fail to recognise it. It is very common for people in their pursuit for happiness, search for it not within themselves but in other people and in material things. Many assume that things such as a good job, more money, better relationships, and others will give them the happiness that they are searching for. That is, until they reach this and do not get what they think they are going to.

My main focus is working on attachment and trauma to help individuals move forward with their life without the replaying of old patterns. For me, getting to the root of what we see is important in the healing process. A lot of the work I do focuses on the inner child. It is here where the secrets to our success and our overall happiness lies, and I absolutely love supporting people during this process of uncovering. I work with the mind and body through the healing process.

Over the several years I have been supporting clients, I have come to realise that the main underlying root cause of the majority of presenting behaviours and unhappiness is often the relationship we hold with ourselves. What do I mean by this? I mean that through our upbringing, we are conditioned. This is no one's fault, but it is the meaning we give to an experience that has happened. We develop an identity of who we are through this conditioning and strive to be what we think we should be. We seek happiness in this conditioned world and become further disconnected from our authentic self.

What is an authentic self? It is the true person you strive to be. We can find ourselves in a place where we don't know how to love ourselves, feeling lost and confused. We become in conflict with what our conditioned self thinks and what our authentic self thinks. The emotions of not following your conditioned self can stop you from being happy. For example, you may want to be a lawyer, but your family wants you to be a doctor, so rather than feel the emotional response of guilt or shame, you do what they want to avoid the emotional sensation. We can learn from all our past experiences to understand the meaning and interpretation we have given to them to understand why we are the way we are.

Ultimately, we can find out what happiness means to you. It's time for you to meet you! It's time for you to put yourself first. This is your life. The secret to reaching your greatness is to communicate with your thoughts and learn to manage your emotions. Oh, and the main ingredient is of course to love who you are!

I am very grateful for what I learn from interacting with others. I am inspired by people's transformations in their personal and professional lives, and it gives me great joy to watch them excel in their health, wealth, relationship, and ultimately, their happiness goals.

Each of us holds unimaginable power within ourselves, a power that is so strong, so extraordinary, and so beautiful, which if you tap into and unleash, it can transform you and your overall   happiness. The way you react has been repeated thousands of times; it becomes comfortable for you to behave this way. To change is to start with awareness and to understand patterns of behaviour.

All of us imagine our ideal life to be a certain way. Some may want a simple life with loved ones around, while others may want more wealth. Each of us strive for happiness in a different way, and that is okay! Happiness is a state of one's mind. We do not look for it. We do not even have to chase it. Happiness, in truth, lies within ourselves, starting from us and ending at us, being self-satisfied.

Happiness is when your life fulfills your needs. You do not feel happiness all the time, but it is a frequent positive emotion you feel. In other words, happiness comes when you feel satisfied and fulfilled. It is a feeling of contentment and joy that life is just as it is. It does not mean that when you are happy you do not feel emotions such as sadness, anxiety, and anger, because you do! A 'happy person' will experience the spectrum of emotions just like anybody else, but the frequency by which they experience the negative ones may differ. Nobody is immune to life's stressors, but the question is whether you see those stressors as moments of opposition or moments of opportunity.

I believe happiness is a choice, that you have the ability to create real and lasting happiness for yourself. Happiness is also related to life satisfaction, appreciation of life, and moments of pleasure, but overall it is to do with how you experience your emotions. After all, it is our emotions that create our reality. Happiness is intangible; you can't put it in your pocket and save it for later. Everyone is different and what qualifies as 'happy' to one person will be different for another. Life circumstances can also affect happiness, such as upbringing, health, and finances.

Growing up, we are conditioned in a way to give meaning to the world around us and seek happiness externally. This is not a blaming game, but to understand why we are the way we are. Happiness creates enjoyable emotions such as contentment, joy, and inner peace. Thus, what we attach or are conditioned to think happiness is, this is what we strive to seek through the external world. The problem with this is we only gain temporary fulfilment. For example, we strive to pass our exams, get a car, get married, have kids, buy our next house, buy those shoes we have had our eyes on, etc. It feels good to have this for a short time… but then what?

Don't wait to be happy. If you only allow yourself to be happy when you hit big life goals, you are missing the bigger picture. It is about your journey and celebrating the little wins, not waiting for huge milestone achievements. Define and give yourself clarity of what winning, success, and happiness means to you on a daily basis—not just at a specific goal.

The secret to your happiness lies inside of you. It is to understand and become consciously aware of your blueprint, your beliefs, and why you see the world the way you do. When we compare ourselves or our happiness with others, it makes us doubt our own path and success. The thing is we all grow at different rates, and that is okay. A rose and a sunflower both need different environments to blossom and flourish, each with its unique beauty.

We do not realise it, but somewhere within us there is a supreme self at peace. The relationship we have with ourselves is one of the most important relationships in life. It sets the tone for all other relationships in life, such as with friends, family, romantic partners, food, money, etc. If you develop the relationship you have with yourself, you develop all other relationships in your life. It is so important to nurture that relationship with yourself to feel happy and at peace.

A person's mind is so powerful. We can invent, create, experience and destroy things with thoughts alone. I have found that in order to feel happiness, we need to be able to have a level of awareness of ourselves. It is to break down what happiness means. For me, happiness is peace. True peace comes from self-love, self-compassion, and striving for self-actualization.

I am always teaching myself:

- To be present in the world where chaos and noise can take over,
- To parenting my child self,
- To forgive people who project their internal world to us,
- To respect perspectives,
- To realise labels placed on myself and others that have given context and meaning,
- To not see it as a criticism, but as an opinion,
- To protecting my energy,
- To creating boundaries,
- To breathe,
- To have fun.

I have always said that life is simple, but it is emotions that can complicate it. The better we get at communicating, the better we become at life. So, remember it is emotions that is the glue to how we see the world around us. Feel the feeling but don't become the emotion. Acknowledge it. Understand it. Release it. Emotions will come and go, and that is okay. Have you ever seen someone take their dog for a walk but actually it is their dog taking them for a walk? That is how our emotions can be. Learn to manage them so you can work with them to go through life, so they don't end up dragging you through your life.

Be yourself. If you water yourself down to please people or to fit in or to not offend anyone, you lose the power, the passion, the freedom, and the joy of being uniquely you. You are loved for just being who you are, just for existing. You don't have to do anything to earn it. Your shortcomings, lack of self-esteem, physical perfection, or social or economic success—none of that matters. You are you. Don't be something you think others want you to be. If you do not like who you are, you may have a hard time accepting others liking you. If you do not trust yourself, you may not believe others should trust you and may find it difficult to trust others. The relationship with self holds power to how you behave with others. Take notes, understand, and make the changes you feel you need; just don't lose yourself trying to be something else for others. Your needs matter! You matter!

Anything that I have been able to accomplish today has been a direct result of the lessons the Universe has offered to me and the opportunities I have taken. This has come from what others have taught me, challenged me to do, supported me through, coached me, and even forced me to accomplish. I thank you and the Universe for letting me have and learn from these lessons.

Life is a journey of self-discovery. The privilege of a lifetime is being who you are. Sometimes you find yourself in the middle of nowhere, and sometimes in the middle of nowhere you find yourself. Be who makes you happy, not what you think will make the world happy.

No matter where you go, you always take yourself with you, so make friends with who you are, give compassion towards yourself, and help yourself on your life journey.
I end this by reminding you that the most vital element to being happy is choice. You can choose to be happy. This comes from developing the relationship you hold with yourself through self-understanding, self-compassion, and self-belief.

Live with intention
Walk to the edge
Listen hard
Practice wellness
Play and laugh
Choose with no regrets
Continue to learn everyday
Appreciate all that is around
Do what you love
Manage emotions
Choose to come from LOVE
Your perception, your reality …
Your happiness.

Let people do what they need to do to make them happy, stay on your path, and you do what you need to do to make you happy.
Simple.
The end.

Love, Joy, and Thank you.

About the Author

Dr. Lalitaa Suglani

Lalitaa's USP is that she teaches "simple steps that produce dramatic and life-changing results." She seamlessly brings her integrative styled therapy techniques to the podium, leaving her clients both transfixed and transformed. She focuses on the emotions, thought patterns, and mental habits that can be detrimental or beneficial to our success.

Her speciality is in attachment and trauma and she brings the Inner Child into the work she does with clients. She believes that for long-lasting change to occur, you need to understand the root. Dr. Suglani has always been fascinated by people's behaviours and what makes people do what they do. She has learnt that our behaviours come from our thoughts, and our thoughts can be influenced by the world around us. She understands that we all feel emotions, and it is these emotions that are fuelled from our thoughts and create the reality that we live.

Lalitaa works with individuals to build emotional and psychological resilience by providing appropriate services tailored to meet their specific needs, as we are all different and require something that fits us.

Her mission is to continue to empower individuals to thrive in life, personally grow, elevate relationships, and to be happy! You deserve to!

Contact Information:
Website: www.DrLalitaa.com
Email: hello@DrLalitaa.com
Instagram: Dr.Lalitaa
Facebook and Linkedin: Dr. Lalitaa Suglani

DR. DIAMOND'S HAPPY BRAIN/ MIND PROTOCOL

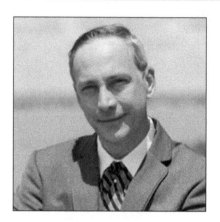

Dr. Michael Diamond

I was neither a healthy nor happy child growing up in a one-bedroom apartment with my parents in the Brooklyn projects in the 1960s and 70s. Being raised by a passive loving father and a two-pack-a-day smoking, hypercritical mother who bed rested me if I had a mere sniffle or earache formed my health patterns for the next several decades. As the old saying goes, "Children learn what they live." As an infant I had colic, then scarlet fever at age three, severe asthma, multiple food allergies, and IBS as a teen and young adult. After becoming a chiropractor in 1990, I usually worked six long days a week. I became run-down and developed chickenpox in 1994, then Lyme CNS and transient myelitis in 1998 which put me out of work, lost 38 pounds from C. diff. as a result of the antibiotics, babesiosis in 2003, measles in 2007, ehrlichiosis in 2009, and Rocky Mountain spotted fever in 2010. As you can see, my immune system was never strong and robust and my nickname as a teen was "Bones."

When I was very young, I was groomed to be a cantor, but at age 13 I decided that I did not want to pursue the religious path. I believe that I gravitated to the healing arts because of my suffering and wanted to help others so that they could feel better about themselves. The many illnesses throughout my life prompted me to immerse myself in nutritional biochemistry, metabolic pathways, exercise physiology, integrative healthcare, and the metaphysics of suffering and healing. I concluded that my mind's perception, interpretation, and internalization of chronic stress played a major role in the weakening of my immune system and development of chronic illnesses, something that went far beyond my genetic enzyme pathway defects.

For most of my teens and young adult life, I lived in a spiritual void. I was a rationalist and reductionist; math and science ruled my existence. What changed my life paradigm and shifted me to a spiritual path was an African violet in the 1990s. I had this plant in my sunroom, and I used to touch its leaves gently, fed it, and watered it periodically. When I got sick with Lyme, my plant got sick as well. I didn't correlate it at the time, but I tried everything to get it better. I changed its food supply, location, water quality, and prayed over it, but the leaves died, and the plant shriveled up. I eventually gave up on it but couldn't throw it out. When my health improved several months later through a holistic treatment program, the plant reanimated and came back to life! I was astounded and it taught me a great life lesson. We are in continuous contact with our environment and what we think and how we feel affects all around us, whether they are in the animal, plant, or mineral kingdoms. This prompted me to immerse myself into holistic health and metaphysics, and I opened up a new branch to my practice in addition to chiropractic care.

When patients present to me for the first time and ask me how they can heal from their particular list of chronic health conditions and transform their life, the first statement I say is that you must try to get your mind in the right place PRIOR to starting any program. Proper mindset is critical for health transformation, followed by the proper treatment plan, guidance, and support.

I will usually ask the patient two simple questions at the

beginning of the interview, but few can answer these questions without a great pause:

1. "Define yourself in one word."
2. "Define happiness," or "Why are you alive?"

After the responses, we set health goals together.

Before we embark on the exciting journey on how to optimally wake up your mind/brain, there are some important concepts to understand:

1. Your **skull** is the chalice for the brain.
2. The **brain** houses the mind. The brain and the mind are NOT the same! The brain is the physical organ that houses the mind and consciousness, and it is the most neglected organ treated in conventional healthcare today.
3. We actually have **three "brains"** that we must control! (This is known as the triune brain theory.) The intellectual center resides in the neocortex and is called the primate "thinking" brain. The emotional center resides in the limbic system (the amygdala and nucleus accumbens), with minicenters in the solar plexus and nervous system, collectively called the mammal "feeling" brain. The instinctual/sexual/motor center resides in the base of the brain (the brainstem and cerebellum), with minicenters in the thoracic spine and the reproductive organs, collectively called the reptilian "instinctive" brain. The reptilian brain is responsible for the 4Fs... fight, flight, feed and fornicate. <u>In order to make these three brains "happy," we must be safe from danger, establish positive social bonds, learn, and be connected to a higher purpose.</u> All three layers of the brain are connected via an extensive network of nerves that influence each other via electrochemical impulses and link emotions with thinking and voluntary actions.
4. Your **mind** is an invisible, interdimensional transmitter/ receiver of consciousness that connects the higher world

(the spiritual realm) to the lower world (the physical realm) via the soul. The mind is not confined to the brain. The mind is where you become aware of your own life. The various intelligences of your mind permeate through every cell of your body, not just your brain cells. When the mind controls the body, you have self-control. When we sleep, our brain shrinks in size to 60% so that it can rid its waste and our mind travels to the astral realm for dreaming, where our laws of physics do not apply. This is why you can fly or do all kinds of superhero stuff in your dreams.

5. **Thoughts** are silent and invisible and occur in the mind. The mind creates thought in another dimension at virtually the speed of light. You must choose your thoughts wisely as recurrent thoughts tend to manifest in physical form. The most important factor in bringing a thought into physical manifestation is the clarity of the visualization.

6. **Neuroplasticity** is the mind's ability to change the structure of our brain matter by forming and reorganizing synaptic connections, especially in response to experience or following injury.

7. **Humans have five basic brain wave patterns and three states of mind.**

The five brain wave patterns are:

1. <u>Delta</u> – dreamless sleep, deep meditation
2. <u>Gamma</u> – process brainwaves simultaneously, modulate perception & spiritual emergence
3. <u>Theta</u> – light sleep, deep meditation
4. <u>Alpha</u> – awake, alert, relaxed
5. <u>Beta</u> – awake, alert, thinking

Our brain waves determine our emotional states, perception, and how we react to external events. Overarousal or underarousal of the waves are linked to mood disorders, insomnia, PTSD, impulsive behaviors, chronic pain syndrome, hypoglycemia, etc. Our three states are mind are the subconscious, the conscious, and the superconscious. Each level of consciousness represents a different intensity of awareness. There are meditations and brain-based therapies that can help to balance your brain waves and cultivate awareness of your three levels of consciousness.

After 30-plus years of accumulating patient data and reviewing research, I have observed five simple concepts that are critical for achieving optimal brain/mind/body health:

1. "What you eat influences your mind. You are what you eat. You are what you think."
2. "Guard your tongue what you say and how you eat."
3. "He who controlleth his blood elements through proper lifestyle, controls his mind.
4. "He who controlleth his mind, controls his words and his deeds."
5. "He, who also controlleth his mind, controls his cells, genes, overall health and ultimately his destiny."

Before you embark on a brain optimization program, you should be tested. In evidence-based healthcare, you test, implement a treatment strategy, obtain patient feedback, and then reassess and refine. Survey forms are initially used to assess how the patient feels about their symptoms and gives us a starting point for treatment. The second step is to use specific laboratory tests to screen, monitor, and adjust their biological terrain. The third step is to perform structural and functional brain tests. The recommended structural test is an MRI of the brain unless there is trauma, and then possibly a CAT scan. I like the NeuroQuant® program, which can be ordered with an MRI. The NeuroQuant® program looks for age-related brain atrophy (Alzheimer's, dementia), hippocampal volume asymmetry (epilepsy), multi-structure atrophy (MS, neurodegenerative conditions), concussion, and PTSD management. There are several functional brain tests that I use to assess general cognitive function (short-term memory, attention span, brain processing speed, and switching of attention). Once you establish your baseline, then you are ready to implement lifestyle changes.

I have broken down my wakeup the brain/mind treatment protocol into five categories:

1. <u>Mental methods</u> – contemplation, visualization, retrospection, introspection, and talk therapy
2. <u>Physical methods</u> – breath work (pranayama), chiropractic care, exercise (stretching, strengthening, cardio), and myofascial release
3. <u>Neurochemical methods</u> – anti-inflammatory diet based upon over 13 quality of life variables, targeted dietary supplementation, and prescription medication (if necessary)
4. <u>Neuroelectrical methods</u> – balancing the five major brain frequencies with specific frequencies of light and sound (neurofeedback), and music therapy
5. <u>Spiritual methods</u> – prayer, meditation, chanting, mantras, mudras, rites and rituals (depending upon your Eastern or Western faith system)

Key Points:

• Imbalances in the spine (vertebral subluxation complexes) can lead to impaired feedback to the brain, which can adversely affect coordination, muscle tone, pain level, movement fluidity, and even mood stability.

• I am personally opposed to using psychedelics for brain optimization or for seeking self-discovery/spiritual enlightenment unless the patient goes to an authentic shaman for the purpose of exiting out of a drug-dependent lifestyle or intractable depression/grief where all traditional methods have failed.

• I have not included the sixth method, energetic medicine, in my protocol as this is not my specialty. However, I believe that it is a vital component of cognitive repair AFTER the first three methods are utilized and in place.

• Patients are free to do as little or as much as they desire depending upon their life schedules, priorities of work or family life, and their comfort zone. Methods #1 and #5 help the mind extend its consciousness beyond the limitations of its physical reality and allow it to experience higher dimensions of consciousness.

• I have found that the more effort you put in the front end early in life (prevention), the less effort you will have to exert later in life in the back end (disease, prescription meds, surgeries).

• Why perform a brain optimization program early in life? Studies have shown that the brain starts to accumulate amyloid plaque about 20 years before the symptoms of Alzheimer's appear.

In order to wake up your brain <u>mentally</u>, you should focus on seven critical goals:

1. "Know thyself," as per the Oracle of Delphi via the ancient disciplines of introspection and retrospection.
2. Accept full responsibility for your thoughts, words, deeds, and life situations via the spiritual path. Learn to keep your word when you make any promises.

The spiritual path = purification of your thoughts, words and deeds

Thoughts	Words	Deeds
Prayer	No yelling, screaming, or cursing	Purification rituals
Meditation	No sarcasm	Drink clean water
Introspection	No blaming others	Eat organic, live foods
Retrospection	Maintain positive speech	Optimize sleep
Cultivate virtues – "angels"		Exercise regularly
Eliminate vices – "demons"		Charity
Develop attitudes of happiness		Have pets and cultivate nature

3. Maintain a balanced lifestyle. Strive for nothing to excess and lead a simple life.
4. Develop and maintain patience, persistence, dedication, and a positive attitude in all of your endeavors.
5. You must repair self-image (how you portray yourself to the world) before repairing self-esteem (how you feel about yourself deep down). Repair self-image first by talking more confidently, improving your daily hygiene habits, wearing nice comfortable clothing, and smiling to the world, even when you don't want to. Appearing to be in control is your first step even though you may not feel that way internally.
6. You must repair your self-esteem next because everything in your life completely revolves around it. Self-esteem is your ability to protect yourself, assert your feelings and take charge. A low self-esteem is a spiritual crisis, not a psychological one. The key to building your self-esteem is simply holding yourself accountable to a realistic standard that you set for yourself, not worrying about what others think and letting go of the critical voices or traumas of the past.
7. The goal when trying to achieve health is not to accumulate vast bits of knowledge, but to find guidance and support and receive wisdom from a healthcare practitioner who has put time into a clinical practice, is willing to listen to you and guide you on the path.

You will know when you have transformed your mind when you achieve mastery of the Self. Mastery of the Self occurs when you appear to have a state of harmony in your life and you have a stable mood, an abundance of energy, you sleep soundly, you start to have a reverence and love for all life, and you appear to be in excellent health and feel happy.

The three harmonies that you must seek and achieve are:

1. Harmony with oneself.
2. Harmony with others.
3. Harmony with nature.

Shifting gears, in order to wake up your brain <u>chemically</u>, you should follow the "4R system," as described in gut restoration programs: remove, replace, reinoculate, and repair.

Remove

1. Reduce daily psychological stressors.
2. Don't smoke or drink alcohol to excess!
3. Get rid of all clutter in the house seasonally. Become a minimalist and not a hoarder.
4. Reduce pathogen load (chronic viruses, bacteria, and fungi).
5. Follow an anti-biofilm protocol since most pathogenic microbes prefer living in biofilm communities for their protection. Biofilms are formed by bacteria attaching to surfaces and forming a protective matrix around them. The biofilm secretes substances that protect the foreign bacteria from our immune systems. Biofilms that are formed in the human body are up to 10,000 times more resistant to antibiotics than free-floating bacteria. This makes biofilm very difficult to treat and explains the persistence of many bacterial infections. Some examples of bacteria hiding in biofilms are otitis media, dental plaque, bacterial endocarditis, chronic Lyme, chronic wounds that do not heal within three months, hospital-acquired infections from catheters, cystic fibrosis, and Legionnaire's disease.
6. Reduce environmental toxins and toxic metal loads via a specific OVERNIGHT toxin removal protocol. WARNING: NEVER detox during the day! Why? The body needs the time during sleep to lower free radical levels, increase master antioxidant concentrations, and to detox, rebuild, and heal. Remember, the brain uses almost as much energy to repair itself while sleeping as in the awake state! Detoxification is best performed for fat- and water-soluble toxin removal in a fasted state at night when your metabolism is dedicated to cellular repair. Detoxification is a parasympathetic-dominant event that naturally occurs overnight, which allows the fats cells to

liberate their toxins. When you detox during the day, the sympathetic nervous system is unnecessarily activated which wastes a lot of energy that is required to detox and heal. Most detox programs suggest forcing the body to do the hard work of detoxification in the daytime, which can lead to more Herxheimer reactions, more daytime fatigue and brain fog, and incomplete detoxification.

Replace

7. Replace the Standard American Diet with a combination of calorie restriction, a ketogenic diet, and fermented foods or a vegetarian diet or a classic Mediterranean diet, depending upon your current health status. Use fad diets only for a short period of time to accomplish a weight loss goal.
8. Replace unhealthy drinks and snacks to healthy ones.

Reinoculate

9. Reset and rebuild the gut microbiome.
10. Supply critical brain micronutrients (vitamins, minerals, amino acids).
11. Improve nerve cell (neuron) and mitochondrial health.

Repair

12. Sleep for five REM cycles, which equates to about 7.5 hours of uninterrupted sleep.
13. Heal impaired gut permeability ("leaky gut").
14. Enhance the brain-gut axis.
15. Restore cell membrane phospholipid health.
16. Optimize the gut-immune-liver axis.
17. Decalcify the brain sand in the pineal gland.
18. Enhance brain microcirculation and take targeted nootropics based upon your cognitive deficits.
19. Boost endogenous stem cells and lengthen DNA telomeres.

20. Do a water fast once per month for spiritual purification and elimination of water-soluble toxins.

I will conclude with a statement that I wrote on December 21st, 2012:

"No 'one' or no 'thing' can make you happy. True happiness occurs when one has controlled the Inner Self, conquered your inner demons and cultivated your ethical character to the highest level possible. You must learn, practice and master the great universal principles from withIN. One must not merely read and accept these principles upon faith. Faith will lead your spiritual path exactly where you were TOLD to follow, which may be somewhere or nowhere. The one who performs the Great Work of self-improvement through time-tested practice of doing no harm to yourself or others, persistence and consistent reflection and purification upon one's thoughts, words and deeds will ascend to the greatest heights."

After 29-plus years of full-time clinical practice and a lifetime of personal experience, I have formulated an online, self-guided, self-paced transformation program. Within this intensive introspective and retrospective program, there are six Academies: Breathe Well, 7 Rays Alchemical Nutrition, Sleep Well, Move Well, Think Well, and Energize Well. We also incorporate the 5 Elements Renewal Program for those with chronic health issues. Within the Think Well Academy is a holistic cognitive repair program consisting of neurocognitive strategies, neurochemical dietary supplement recommendations, and a list of meditations and neuroelectrical devices to help balance and harmonize the major brain waves to enhance mood, attention span, short-term memory, brain processing speed, and switching of attention.

For more information, please visit
www.DiamondIntegrativeHealth.com/CRP
The password for the protected document is Nosceteipsum.

I wish you good luck on your health journey!

About the Author

Dr. Michael R Diamond, M.S., D.C.

- Dr. Diamond was born in Brooklyn, NY and received his Bachelor of Science in Athletic Training from Brooklyn College in 1984, his Master of Science in Exercise Physiology from Western Illinois University in 1985, and his Doctor of Chiropractic from New York Chiropractic College in 1990.
- Dr. Diamond has practiced alternative and complementary healthcare since 1991 in Patchogue, New York City, and the Hamptons. He has worked with diverse patient populations ranging from homeless to billionaires, from laborers to Wall Street executives, from junior to elite athletes, and has toured worldwide with music artists and entertainers as their doctor/personal trainer/nutrition counselor/life coach.
- He is a Diplomate, Fellow, and Board Certified in Integrative Medicine from the American Association of Integrative Medicine, certified as a Holistic Health Counselor from the Institute of Integrative Nutrition, and is a graduate of Functional Medicine University.
- Since 1979, Dr. Diamond has extensively studied the physical, chemical, and emotional aspects of holistic healthcare. His interests include exercise physiology, personal training and injury prevention, optimal nutrition and dietary supplementation, thyroid dysfunction, adrenal gland insufficiency, autoimmune disorders, chronic tick-borne illness, neurotransmitter imbalances, hormone replacement therapy, anti-aging and longevity medicine, the metaphysics of chronic illness, and the mindset for radiant health and wellness.
- He is a certified ISSA Master Personal Trainer, First Degree Black Belt in American Jiu Jitsu, certified NESTA Muay Thai fitness coach, certified NESTA Core Conditioning Specialist, and has been Medical Director for the Empire State Karate Nationals and Ringside Doctor for WPKO Pro/Am Kickboxing.
- Dr. Diamond's treatment modalities in complementary and alternative healthcare include:

1. Using safe, evidence-based chiropractic treatment methods to decrease pain, increase range of motion, and improve posture
2. Teaching patients how to move better through progressive functional movement corrective exercise programs (static stretching, dynamic mobility drills, cardio, and strength training)
3. Rebuilding the body from the cellular level up for those with chronic illnesses
4. Balancing the important biochemical pathways through the practice of evidence-based holistic healthcare

5. Developing customized nutrition and weight loss programs to improve body composition (loss of pounds and inches)
6. Naturally correcting neurotransmitter (serotonin, dopamine, norepinephrine, epinephrine, GABA, etc.) imbalances which create a cycle of abnormal eating patterns, (i.e., binge eating, boredom eating, emotional eating, night eating), and mood disorders
7. Recommending mind-body techniques (prayer, meditation, and religious devotion) and brain-based activities to positively alter brain electrical function, mood, and human physiology

Contact Information:
Michael R. Diamond, M.S., D.C.
Diamond Integrative Health, LLC
440 Waverly Ave, suite 4
Patchogue, NY 11772

Telephone: 1-631-758-7111
Email: DrDsfcc@optonline.net

PRACTICAL THINGS YOU NEED TO KNOW ABOUT ANTIAGING REJUVENATIVE MEDICINE AND YOUR BRAIN

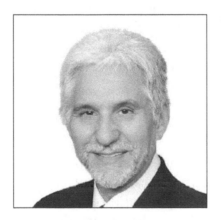

Dr. Michael J Grossman, MD

Youthful aging requires maintaining a chain of many links. If any link is weak and breaks, your goal of youthful aging has failed. Your weakest link is what you need to focus on as you read through this comprehensive description for how to reverse aging. As an antiaging regenerative specialist practicing since 1976, I will tell you what you need to know about reversing aging and keeping your brain young. These are facts and strategies that your doctor may or may not tell you.

Bioidentical Hormone Replacement

Research has become clear that bio-identical hormone replacement for menopausal women and andropausal men extends life, reduces cancer and heart disease, and maintains youthful enthusiasm. Bioidentical hormones improve mood, sleep, brain clarity, enthusiasm, muscle stamina and libido. As men and women age into their 40s and 50s, they need to have blood tests and/or urine and saliva tests to measure hormone levels of estrogen, progesterone, and testosterone in women; testosterone and estrogen in men; and DHEA and growth hormone levels (IGF-I) in both men and women.

For women, replacement hormones for estrogen and testosterone should be topical, injectable, or pellets placed under the skin to reduce unwanted metabolites from oral tablets. Progesterone can be topical or oral. In men, testosterone should be topical, injectable, or pellets placed under the skin. Men will need some kind of prescription estrogen aromatase inhibitor such as anastrozole.

Early Detection of Artery Hardening

Knowledge of artery hardening and thickening is essential as cholesterol levels are poorly correlated with clogging of the arteries. A variety of measurements for arterial stiffness are available for very early detection of artery clogging. CT scans of the coronary arteries are also an early detector. Ultrasound of the carotid arteries can measure intimal thickness, which is also very early detection. Traditional ultrasound of the carotid arteries will only measure actual clogging after there is about 20% to 30% clogging. Traditional treadmill studies are very late and will only detect a problem when there is at least 50% clogging already.

Inflammation

This is a big risk factor for aging, clogging of the arteries, cancer, arthritis and autoimmune disease. Inflammation is caused by a variety of factors but often overlooked is imbalances in the gastrointestinal tract. We can measure a number of inflammatory markers particularly, C-reactive protein-highly sensitive, is a simple blood test. Reducing this inflammatory marker may require an integrated approach of nutritional, herbal, and gastrointestinal probiotic balancing treatments.

Prediabetes

This is a huge risk factor for aging in general and especially your brain specially. You need to know your hemoglobin A1c blood test which should be below 5.7. Above 6.0 is what I consider to be early diabetes. Additionally, it is important to test your fasting insulin blood levels. Below 5.0 is good. If you're between 5 and 20, you need to work with your physician to change your diet and take various herbs and nutrients. An insulin level greater than 20 is diabetes.

Research for longevity and reducing heart disease and stroke indicate that your blood pressure should be below 130/80.

Reversing Aging Body Parts with Stem Cells

I have written a book, *The Magic of Stem Cells: Activating Your Own Healing Power*, which describes the miracle of using our own stem cells to restore, rejuvenate, and repair injured or damaged body parts. Eighty percent of the time, the results are seemingly miraculous.

Repair of injured body parts starts out with your own blood and platelets which create a clot and then release growth factors to call in repair cells. We were very efficient at doing this when we are young, but less efficient when we get older. We can use your own platelet growth factors very simply through a process where we do a blood test and concentrate these growth factors and inject them back into the injured body parts. This works well for minor injuries and gives you six weeks of ongoing repair. The results are quite permanent.

The next step up would be to use stem cells from your own body fat. Stem cells in body fat are like sleeping firemen waiting to be activated to initiate the repair process. Stem cells are very abundant in fat and very easy to obtain through a simple lipo-suction process. Stem cells can be injected locally or intravenously. Intravenous injections will go all over the body including the brain. I have been doing this for over five years with 80% of people having miraculous results. Stem cells and growth factors are also available from the umbilical cord of newborn babies.

Reversing Sexual Dysfunction in Men and Women

Fifty percent of men can expect sexual dysfunction by the time they reach 50 to 60 years of age. Use of Viagra and Cialis are widespread and neutral for reversing the underlying causes of sexual dysfunction but give you some short-term benefit. We now have several approaches that actually reverse the underlying damage that occurs from aging: The P-shot and Gainswave.

The P-shot is platelet rich plasma (PRP) injected directly into the penis to activate repair and rejuvenation just like you might inject PRP into any body part. Gainswave is an acoustic vibrational intense wave that also stimulates the body to repair and rejuvenate. Both approaches work 80% of the time in my experience of many hundreds of patients over the last four years. This also works for Peyronie's disease, which is a curvature of the penis that occurs from bending damage when the penis is not firm enough during intercourse.

A huge problem for women as they reach their 40s and 50s is decreased sensation and decreased ability to experience orgasm. Injecting the vaginal area with platelet rich plasma is known as the O-shot. This is a simple office procedure that has a profound effect on reversing sexual dysfunction in women.

In both men and women, bioidentical hormones are an essential part of restoring youthful sexual functioning.

Skin Aging

This is a big problem that now has a variety of rejuvenative approaches. My favorite is the CO2 pro-fractional laser, which removes 5% your skin with microscopic pinholes in each postage stamp area of your skin. When applied to the whole face, the body repairs these little pinholes with youthful, healthy skin and brings growth factors naturally to your face. We can add additional growth factors topically during the healing process to restore and create skin that looks 10 years younger. The benefits last for many years.

Much of skin aging is caused by loss of youthful fat and bone volume. We can inject materials which stimulate the body's own repair process to regrow collagen in areas that have lost volume. These benefits, depending upon the material used, can last for many years.

Sleep Quality Affects Longevity

Sleep apnea occurs as we get older. When our throat elasticity decreases and breath cannot flow out, we wake ourselves up. Although we may or may not experience interrupted sleep, there is in fact a disruption of the dreaming cycle of REM sleep. This causes daytime sleepiness, high blood pressure, and heart disease. Snoring during the night can be a signal that there may be sleep apnea. In order to properly diagnose this problem, you need to have a sleep apnea screen, which can be done in your home with a sensor on your finger measuring your oxygen levels as you sleep.

In addition, as we get older, we naturally do not sleep as deeply because we don't have as many dreams. This leads to brain degeneration over the years. We can restore youthful sleep by using growth hormone releasing peptides. These peptides naturally release growth hormone that is stored in the pituitary gland. Additional benefits of these peptides are increased muscle stamina, muscle strength, endurance, and loss of body fat.

Relationships

The most important measure of longevity after the age of 50 is the quality of your relationships. The most overlooked and biggest cause of aging as we get to the age of 50 is the quality of your relationships in general, and importantly, your romantic relationship. A remarkable 80-year study called the George Valiant Harvard Study of Longevity showed that whether you come from a poor neighborhood or you are part of the elite Harvard College graduate population, the quality of your romantic relationship is by far the most important measure associated with living longer.

My wife and I have written a book called *The Marriage Map: Transforming Your Marriage from Ordeal to Adventure*. Marriage is not designed to be an easy, smooth experience. It is a process that will promote growth and pressure you to gain skills and wisdom over a lifetime. In our book, we describe how we have had three different marriages. We were 20 and 21 when we married, and we did whatever I thought was best. My wife was very accommodating. In the second marriage, we were in our 30s and my wife went back to graduate school to complete her PhD in the field of marriage and family therapy.

She was no longer as accommodating as she then had the confidence of her own point of view about things. My wife pressed me to be more emotionally present, as well as open and honest. That was a difficult five-year process for us. We went to many classes, courses, and personal development programs during that time. We learned skills to support two independent, autonomous people in becoming emotionally present with each other and accepting of our differences. We learned how to support each other and heal the wounds of our childhood.

Having grown beyond the power struggle and reconnecting at a deeper emotional level, we turned our attention to teaching other couples the skills that we found make the biggest difference in developing partnership in a romantic relationship. For the last 25 years, we have impacted thousands of couples by teaching skills to make requests nicely, to listen deeply to each other without interrupting, to support the healing of each other's childhood wounds, and to stay emotionally and sensually connected to each other.

This impacts the aging process greatly as it changes your emotional, hormonal, and spiritual development. Focusing on happiness alone is not as helpful. Rather, focusing on deep emotional connection and expanding your own ability to love, understand, and appreciate your partner is what creates longevity. These skills will apply to everyone in your life. Generally, after a man has attained competence and success in his business and career, he needs to grow and develop his heart in his ability to forgive and emotionally connect.

In our book, *The Marriage Map*, we tell the story of Percival, the great knight of King Arthur's court, and how he goes through this process, which is a metaphor for what every man needs to do. He first works hard to become the greatest knight in the world. Then, he is magically brought into the Grail castle, which is under a spell. Everyone is waiting for a great knight to come in and ask the suffering king a question that comes from the heart, "What ails thee?" But Percival has been taught that a good knight does not ask questions; rather, he should wait for someone to ask him questions. Thus, he does not come from his heart, but rather from social convention.

He fails in the quest to gain the Holy Grail. It takes him some six years of emotional suffering, introspection, and spiritual mentoring. Finally, he moves into forgiveness and letting go of social conventions in favor of his authentic self. Eventually, he returns the Grail castle and asks the question from his heart, thereby achieving the Holy Grail and becomes the new Grail King. This is the story of every man's journey—if he is willing to go the distance.

The quintessential myth of the female journey is the story of Psyche and Eros (Cupid). Psyche is a beautiful goddess who gives up her goddess-hood to come down to earth to become a woman. Eros falls in love with her but makes her promise never to look at his face except in the dark of night. They are happily married, but when she looks at him one night with a candle, he is upset that she has broken her promise and he leaves. (Women often demand more emotional intimacy than what a man can provide.)

Psyche goes on a long journey of many adventures where she gains great skills and abilities to define her desires, deal with male anger, deepen and strengthen her own personality, and to control her speech and actions. She then becomes an equal to Eros and she rejoins him as a goddess.

In our modern culture, many women now take the path of the Percival journey and learn competence and career success and then learn later to develop the heart and create intimate connection with others. The process of growing in a romantic partnership not only creates longevity but also develops the personality, provides meaning, and fulfills a spiritual purpose of life.

The Best Exercise for Brain Youthfulness

Research is very clear that ballroom dancing is the best exercise for brain rejuvenation and prevention of dementia. The

21-year study of senior citizens 75 and older was published in the *New England Journal of Medicine*. The reduction in dementia was 76% in the frequent dancing group compared to reading (35%), bicycling and swimming (0%), doing crossword puzzles at least four days a week (47%), and playing golf (0%).

There are many exercises that help cardiovascular health and they all have a value. However, ballroom dancing has been shown to be dramatically more effective than any other exercise for maintaining brain youthfulness. This is because ballroom dancing includes physical exercise and involves many different movements coordinated both with the music and your partner. The intense brain activity and muscle coordination involved maintains brain youthfulness. It is far better than crossword puzzles or playing various board games as it combines both the physical and mental qualities of coordination. There is also the additional benefit of pleasurable physical connection with your partner.

My wife and I have the joy of dancing and competing in waltz, tango, foxtrot and quickstep. There are at least 30 things to be mindful of at the same time while we are engaging in dynamic exercise. Reversing aging can be a fun project.

Meditation is Foundational for Health, Creativity, and Longevity

Research on meditation is shown to have a direct correlation with reduced illness, lower blood pressure, less heart disease, less infections, and reduced anxiety and depression. I have taught meditation since 1973 to thousands of individuals. When taught correctly, meditation is easy to learn and profoundly helpful for calmness, psychological health, and personal spiritual growth. There are many excellent practices of meditation. I personally teach deep but easily learned meditation online. You can learn about meditation, relationship courses, and my medical services online at www.OCWellness.com & www.TheMarriageMap.com

In summary, you are as healthy and youthful as your weakest link. My review of the elements involved in taking care of your health with a view towards healthy aging and longevity should give you a blueprint for how to take care of yourself in this new era of anti-aging and rejuvenative medicine.

About the Author

Dr. Michael J Grossman, MD

Dr. Grossman has been specializing in integrative medicine since 1976. His been a pioneer in bioidentical hormone therapy, stem cell therapy, meditation, and antiaging medicine. His office is in Irvine, California.

He is the author of three books: *The Vitality Connection: 10 Practical Ways to Optimize Health and Reverse the Aging Process*, *The Marriage Map: The Road to Transforming Your Marriage from Ordeal to Adventure*, and *The Magic of Stem Cells: Awakening Your Own Healing Power*.

Contact Information:
Website: www.OCWellness.com
Telephone: (949) 222-0232

Information about our *Falling in Love Forever* classes is available at www.themarriagemap.com

YOU JUST NEVER KNOW

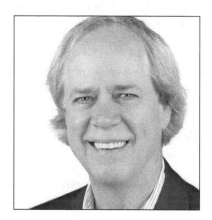

Dr. Reed Moeller DC

My story of success starts with a healthy brain, positive attitude, being grateful for life; always making the best of the circumstance by knowing that what happens is meant to happen. Some of the toughest lessons that happen turn out to be blessings. God and the power of our Universe put people in our lives for a purpose. If we realize events that happen are meant to be, you can learn, grow, and be grateful.

Two of the biggest lifechanging events in my life occurred unexpectedly. Great things happen when you're not looking. These experiences have given me the wisdom to have faith that things will always work out.

The first life-changing event was meeting the love of my life, Kathy. It was the summer of '78 and I worked as a dock boy at the Chicago Yacht Club. My responsibilities were helping boats dock, selling gas, ice, and refreshments. Kathy was waitressing inside the restaurant. She was a drop-dead gorgeous ballerina with very long, blonde hair—totally out of my league. She seemed shy and kept to herself. Working on the docks, I met a lot of the sailboat owners and they would often invite me to go sailing when I got off work. To be social, I would invite coworkers to come along. I always asked Kathy, but she would decline.

It was the summer between my freshman and sophomore year of college at Ohio University and I was still dating my high school sweetheart back home. Needless to say, I wasn't looking to date anyone. I later learned Kathy had been dating a guy in Chicago for several years and wasn't interested in dating anyone else either.

As luck would have it, (or should I say fate) on the final weekend of the summer (two days before I flew back to school), I was having lunch at the club and Kathy waited on me. There was a wine tasting party I was invited to that night in town and even though I expected her to decline and make up a lame excuse, I invited her anyway. She thought about it and by the time I was done eating she surprised me and said, "Yes, pick me up at my father's apartment." I later found out her boyfriend had left for a weekend camping trip and she thought getting out of the house and that going to a party would be fun. She was supposed to go on that camping trip but had to work that weekend.

I was with both of my brothers, so the three of us picked her up and headed the party. At the party we had a great time, and great conversation until I burned her brand-new, leather purse on the stove. I leaned against the knob in the crowded kitchen turning on the burner by accident. We put out the fire, but I felt terrible. I wasn't off to a good start. She was really sweet about it, but I wanted to make it up to her and take her out on a real date… without my brothers! I had one more night in town and she agreed to give me one more shot.

I took her to Benihanas, a Japanese Steak House where you sit at a communal table. It was a fun place with good food and no pressure. Man, did we hit it off! It was like we had known each other for years. We shared amazing conversation and great energy. I never wanted the night to end. The original plan was to go to a movie, but we ended up going back to the harbor and spending the evening on a luxury boat. It was the best night of my life.

I left for college the next day. We both broke up with our

longtime girlfriend/boyfriend and carried on a long-distance relationship for four years minus the summers we spent together. We exchanged countless handwritten love letters and made long-distance phone calls. We were married in 1982, just before starting Chiropractic College. She's been my loving bride for 36 years now.

What are the chances I happened to eat at the club that day, on the last weekend of the summer, and she happened to wait on me, her boyfriend happened to be gone camping, there happened to be a party that night, and she decided to say yes? It was divine intervention. What happens is meant to happen.

The second biggest lifechanging event occurred when I severely injured my low back in college. It was my senior year of pharmacy school at Ohio Northern University and I was the captain of the wrestling team. I was 158 pounds and was messing around at practice, taking on my buddy who wrestled in the 185-pound weight class. I remember shooting in for a double leg takedown and felt a pop with sudden excruciating low back pain that radiated down my left leg. I couldn't stand, sit, or walk without severe pain.

As a pharmacist, the only way I knew to treat pain was through medicine. I was on the strongest pain medications, muscle relaxers, and anti-inflammatories but nothing phased the pain. X-rays and an MRI demonstrated a severe herniated disc at the L5/S1 level. I did physical therapy, massage, and received epidural shots. All the doctors told me the only thing that's going to help is major back surgery.

I thought it was the only thing left to do. My coach was the one that recommended chiropractic. He told me, "What do you have to lose? Once you have surgery, your wrestling career is over." I was nervous and in so much pain. Did I really want someone to crack and pop my back? I thought, *I'm already considering surgery so why not try it?*

I went to the chiropractor. He examined my back, looked at my x-ray, and felt he could help me. He laid me on my side and made a quick thrust on my injured area. It popped and when I got up, I felt almost 80% improvement. I could stand straight and walk without pain. What the heck just happened? How could

I feel so good so fast? Why didn't any of my medical doctors recommend this? This should have been the first thing I did. I went from not being able to walk to wrestling three weeks later.

Right away, I looked into going to Chiropractic College. That's when I decided this was my calling. I wanted to heal people naturally without dangerous drugs and surgery. I wanted to tell people what happened to me and how our bodies have the ability to heal themselves. Stimulating the spine wakes up the brain and turns on the life force that heals the body. Drugs and surgery are dangerous and may cause further damage. Have you ever really listened to those drug commercials? It is better to fix the problem than mask the pain. The key is our brain and nervous system. It all starts there.

I had a patient that was suffering with Crohn's disease. She came to me after falling out of a truck and injuring her low back. Much like my condition, she had a badly herniated a disc in her low back, causing back pain down her left leg. She was told she needed back surgery and was out of work.

While treating her back condition, she told me about her digestive issues and how she's had stomach pain after every meal for 20 years. She has had multiple surgeries to remove inflamed sections of her colon. She lived on steroids and pain medication. That is why she couldn't take any more medication for her back. I suggested while we were treating her back condition, we could do acupuncture treatments, BrainTap, and put her on a nutritional program for her Crohn's.

Acupuncture, much like chiropractic, is all about energy, and channels it to where the body needs healing. My acupuncture instructor explained it as fine-tuning the frequency on your radio to make the station come in clearer by getting rid of the static.

BrainTap is an amazing technology to calm and balance the brain. You simply wear headphones and eye covers, and then you close your eyes. All you have to do is relax and the device takes care of the rest. It is like a forced meditation that clears the subconscious of all the negative thoughts and stress, getting your brain into a healing state. It uses light, sound, and a meditative voice; it's magic. We use it while the patient is getting acupuncture and most of the time, they fall asleep.

I treated her twice a week for six weeks (which is the standard protocol for acupuncture). Her back healed through treatment and she returned to work. She came back in after a couple of months for a maintenance adjustment and was so excited. She was almost in tears telling me her Crohn's disease was gone. She was off all her meds and could eat again without suffering pain. Her GI specialist could not believe what he was seeing. She said the only thing she did differently was the acupuncture. It did the job! Some credit has to go to the chiropractic, BrainTap, and the nutritional program we had her on.

She has been healthy now for several years. What an amazing feeling to change someone's life! Once again, she had a terrible back injury that surprisingly led to curing her Crohn's disease. She was in the right place at the right time. You just never know where life will lead and what twists and turns will direct you to the right path.

I wish more people knew and trusted in natural healing. Instead, they choose instant symptom relief by popping a pill whether there are dangerous side effects or not. Pain is a normal response. It is an alarm telling us there is a problem that needs care. If we numb or block that signal and ignore the cause of the pain, the condition will continue to deteriorate. It's kind of like placing tape over our engine light and not fixing the engine. Our bodies are intricate machines that need proper maintenance, but maintenance takes effort. I have a sign in my office that says, "If you don't take care of your body, where are you going to live?" The older we get, the more important our health becomes. Be proactive and take care of it now. Don't be afraid to get a chiropractic adjustment.

I had a spouse of a patient who saw her get better with chiropractic but was afraid to be adjusted and opted for back surgery instead. He would rather have anesthesia, get cut open and drilled upon, risking the dangers of infection and medication before going through a period of painful rehabilitation. Maybe it's that popping sound that I was originally scared of. Years later, he is finally seeing me because he doesn't want to have to go through another surgery—and he won't because he's doing great and loves getting adjusted.

The bottom line is our bodies have the ability to heal and regenerate. It starts with our brain and nervous system and its connection with the heart and gut that controls and regulates everything. These are important structures to take care of. Everything runs through the brain, so let's start controlling our thoughts and reducing our stress by taking care of our brain and spine.

Another case study I am proud of was a teenage girl who had suffered with horrific migraines for years. Her daily headaches were so bad she had to live in the dark and was constantly sick. She had to be homeschooled because it was next to impossible for her to concentrate at times. This girl was on strong medication that had been changed several times due to its ineffectiveness. She was depressed and suicidal. Her mom had been a patient and she asked if I could help.

Obviously, what she was doing wasn't working, and I am used to being considered as the last resort. Of course I knew combining chiropractic, acupuncture, BrainTap, myofascial release, and nutrition would help her recover. What else could be better than relaxing the brain, improving the brain-body connection, balancing the energy in the body, breaking up chronic muscle tension, and healing the gut?

They were all-in and after several months she was headache-free and enrolled back in regular school. She was socially active for the first time in years. This patient ended up going to college and her headaches are now a distant memory. Never lose hope because you just never know.

As a side note, a funny thing happened, her mom told me that Children's Hospital contacted her and said she qualified for a trial of an experimental drug and she should come in and start taking this right away. Her mom told them she doesn't have headaches anymore, yet they suggested she take it anyway because of her history of chronic headaches. Unbelievable. "Let's just take this experimental drug anyway, no matter the consequence."

This is what we are up against. Big Pharma wants to name it and tame it with medication. Forget about doing the things to get healthy and making those lifestyle changes necessary to treat the underlying cause. It's what we all need to do because disease is preventable, and it is my lifelong mission to teach and preach what it takes.

Life is good for me. I have a happy marriage, homelife, and a job where I have the opportunity to change people's lives and prevent them from a lifetime of suffering. Chiropractic miracles occur all the time and nothing is more rewarding to see and be part of it. It requires having a healthy mindset, trusting the Universe and Mother Nature that we have the ability to heal if we just take care of ourselves. Let go of the past, live in the present, and stop worrying about the future. Every day, every season, and every year is a new beginning. Let it be.

About the Author

Dr. Reed Moeller, DC

Dr. Moeller owns and treats patients at the Forest Park Chiropractic & Acupuncture Center in Cincinnati, Ohio. He's committed to caring for each patient like they are family and strives to be the best doctor in his field.

Dr. Moeller graduated from Ohio Northern University and went on to receive his doctorate from Texas Chiropractic College. Dr. Moeller opened Forest Park Chiropractic in 1989. Thirty years later, the practice is still going strong in the very same location.

In 2009, Dr. Moeller graduated from the International Academy of Medical Acupuncture and passed his board exams to become licensed to practice acupuncture in Ohio. Acupuncture and chiropractic care combine to provide the best treatment for ailing bodies, helping to improve the way the body functions in order to allow it to heal itself naturally.

Contact Information:
Forest Park Chiropractic and Acupuncture
1250 W. Kemper Rd.
Cincinnati, OH 45240
Telephone: (513) 742-0880
Email: fpchiro@yahoo.com

THE POWER OF THE BRAIN FOR OPTIMAL HUMAN PERFORMANCE

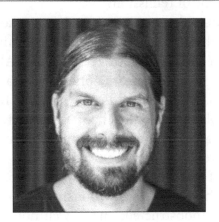

Dr. Noah J Moos

Picture this, you are at your peak physical condition and are an athlete running in the ultimate competition, the Olympics. You are neck and neck with all your competitors, and you are approaching the finish line fast. Your legs are tired but suddenly, in a split second, you are able to dig deep and ignite another gear, and before you know it you, are blowing past everyone, breaking the tape, getting first place, and achieving a lifelong dream. This is the epitome of mastering human potential. Now picture yourself the next season, starting to develop one injury after the next. You experience joint pain that won't go away, and your body doesn't perform as it used to. Unfortunately, this is a common scenario. Athletes often plateau and decline in their performance. Most people chalk it up to getting older. What if I told you this didn't have to happen, and you can maintain longevity in your sport?

Now I want you picture yourself as a 35-year-old mother of two. You've just had your second child and you work a very stressful demanding job in the city. You start to feel weak and are frightened at the feeling of tingling and numbness in both your legs. Walking becomes increasingly difficult. You are no longer able to perform the same activities you've done for years. On top of all that, it's now a struggle to pick up and carry your children. After a trip to the doctor, you are diagnosed with MS (multiple sclerosis). You now feel helpless and are worried about your future. What if I told you there are ways to reset your health and have the hope of remission?

I've encountered these situations in my practice plus many more. While these situations may be seemingly unrelated, they illustrate a common truth at their core. All these patients experienced a breakdown in brain, neural, and cellular communication. In other words, the message from their brain played a terrible game of telephone where the message got distorted with each level of communication until the message became incoherent and unrecognizable.

In the next part, I explain how these patients regained their health. Their recovery demonstrates the importance of a healthy, fast, unobstructed, and a well-nourished brain and neural communication system. I use these same principles to treat everyone from elite athletes to chronically ill patients. Fundamental knowledge has universal roots, and these principles can be applied to heal across many conditions, allowing you to reach your human potential and heal from what seems impossible.

Our body is electric, and our brain and nerves work together with our muscles like a breaker box in a house. Breaker boxes are designed to distribute the appropriate amount of electrical current to different parts of the home. Each section of the home can handle a certain amount of electricity; too little and appliances will not work, too much and you cause the main breaker to trip and you have a power outage.

Our body works the same way. Each muscle and tissue have a certain load it can handle. When each pathway is optimized, it can generate the maximum amount of force and energy and has an increased resistance to fatigue and injury. This allows athletes to perform their sport to the highest potential and chronically ill patients to navigate infection, toxicity, and inflammation. To effectively communicate, the brain and nervous system signals must be clear and uninterrupted. Essentially, we need healthy breakers and the ability to hit reset when things get out of hand.

So what are the types of things that can overload the breakers in muscles and tissues? Chronic levels of structural, chemical, and emotional stress are the main culprits. Structural stress can be anything physically demanded by our body, whether it's working out or an outright injury. Chemical stress can be the result of a poor or unbalanced diet, infections, and environmental toxicity. Emotional stress is something we all deal with, whether we want to admit it or not. So how do all these things affect our body?

Every movement must be processed via the nerves in our nervous system; from the brain to the tissues, and back from the tissues to the brain. The speed, amplitude, and velocity at which this pathway works is of the utmost importance in health and performance. When a college athlete is asked, "What is the difference between college and the pros?" They answer, "The speed of the game." What they mean is the speed at which the brain can process information. When our brain, nerves, and muscles are healthy, they can handle and organize a lot of information quickly and efficiently. When the brain is inflamed, impaired, and bogged down from excessive stressors, the message that needs to be delivered is much slower and may be too late. With these stressors, an athlete may not have the neural efficiency to assimilate the information they need to catch a ball at the right moment, switch to another speed during a race, or react to an incoming punch. These stressors can also cause dysregulation in the function of the immune system, organs, and body tissues in someone who is chronically ill.

As we accumulate unresolved physical, chemical, and emotional stress, the efficiency of the body plummets. It is very similar to a congested freeway with lots of stop-and-go traffic; things move slower. And what often happens on a congested freeway? There's always that one guy who's in too big of a hurry and then crashes into someone else, shutting down the entire freeway. Injuries happen in a similar way. As our body gets congested, there is often a trigger that overloads the body and causes a 'wreck.' Oftentimes the trigger is so small it would normally not cause any type of injury to the body, but the body is too overloaded and cannot deal with it properly.

The overload becomes even more complicated because as humans we have an amazing ability to adapt. If a wreck happens, we reroute. But after so many wrecks, traffic comes to a standstill and we are not able to make any more progress along our route. To get to where we need to go, we now have to go off-road because the freeway is shut down, but our car isn't designed for that terrain and it gets damaged and breaks down. This is when degeneration happens. Our tissues break down because they can no longer handle the load placed upon them.

Degeneration is where we meet our Olympic athlete and MS patient. Both have been pushing the envelope for years. Each have been exposed to large amounts of physical, chemical, and emotional stress for years and their body has adapted and allowed them to push forward to achieve great things, but both have now hit a point where their bodies are failing to adapt to their current stress load. Their freeways are congested, and their breakers are blown. When you examine these patients, it's not uncommon to see the same patterns. I know it's crazy to think, "How can an Olympic athlete and MS patient have similar findings?" But when we consider the fundamental principles of brain, neural, and cellular communication, it's easy to make the connection.

How do we address this breakdown in brain, neural, and cellular communication? Our body has a number of built-in healing pathways, that when stimulated, not only help our body perform better but can improve our immune response, allow our organs to function better, and help us feel more energetic and happier. Let's take some time to look at all these amazing pathways our body has and how we can utilize them for healing. These pathways are our nervous system, meridian system, neurovascular system, and neurolymphatic system. Notice that most all of these are connected back through the brain.

The Nervous System: The Brain, Spinal Cord, and Nerves

Let's start with the master switch: the brain, spinal cord, and nerves. These structures have influence over every organ, tissue, and muscle in the body. If there is interference or inflammation affecting any of these communication pathways, it can have a profound effect on how the body functions.

What if I told you that by stimulating one area of your spine, you could double or triple the pounds per square inch of force your arms and legs exert? This happens when you remove interference and inflammation from the spine, allowing for a more powerful and direct line of communication without interruption. When we have a fixation in any level of the spine, it creates an inflammatory response. This leads to less output by the muscles creating weakness, less ability for the body to adapt to stress, sluggish functioning of the organs, and eventually disease and degeneration. To clear these fixations in the body and reopen communication, I use chiropractic care with my patients.

In addition to chiropractic care, I use a technique called Quantum Neurology Rehabilitation. It has been one of the greatest and most profound techniques for addressing neurologic deficits. Quantum Neurology is an amazing neurologic rehabilitation technique that combines light therapy with specific physical corrections to enhance the communication of the nervous system and brain. What many people do not realize is that our nerves are fiber optic, meaning they transmit and receive light for communication. Amazingly you can use light to reorganize neural patterns. Quantum Neurology has been used to help restore everything from severe neurologic deficits to optimizing the performance of the best athletes in the world. Therefore, it is our treatment of choice when it comes to optimizing and reorganizing nervous system function.

The Meridian System

The meridian system is perhaps the oldest of all the healing systems we have today, as it's rooted in the ancient practice of Chinese medicine. Just like the nervous system, it is a robust information highway, but this one has different routes and connections. In Chinese medicine there the 12 meridians (highways) that are named after organs in the body. Each meridian is also related to different muscles, nutrients, emotions, and times of the day and year. We can measure the output of these meridians to see if energy is high, low, normal, or unbalanced. These patterns of energy output can give us information about underlying causes of injury and illness in the body. We can analyze the meridians to decode things like hidden infections, food sensitivities, allergies, toxic exposure, electromagnetic pollution, and environmental pollution. We can heal by removing the harmful substances or infections from our environment and balancing the meridians using acupuncture, meridian-specific nutrition, and resolving associated emotions. When we learn to read and interpret the meridian system, we can gather a plethora of information that can quickly give us direction for restoring our health.

Neurovascular and Neurolymphatic System

The last two information highways I want to talk about are the circulatory system and the lymphatic system. Our circulatory system pumps blood throughout the body to deliver oxygen, nutrition, and hormones. Our lymphatic system uses lymph to drain inflammatory and immune byproducts from our tissues to help eliminate toxins and waste from the body. We want to make sure each organ, muscle, and tissue in the body has proper blood flow and lymph drainage.

How do we do this? There are reflexes all over our body that can be used to stimulate our brain to increase lymph drainage and blood flow to certain areas. These points are called neurovascular and neurolymphatic reflex points. These built in ancient reflexes allow us to reconnect our brains to our blood vessels and lymphatic channels.

It's fantastic because we can gather more information about the body by testing these reflexes. When an organ, muscle, or tissue is congested because of too much lymph or lack of blood flow, oftentimes these reflexes will be very tender. Stimulating these tender spots have been shown to increase the circulation to different organs, muscles, and tissue using an imaging technique called fluoroscopy. When you increase circulation and lymph drainage, you can start to provide great relief from chronic pain, inflammation, and swelling.

In closing, let's check back in with our Olympian and mother.

Our Olympian's biggest problem is they were a master of adaptation. This sounds like a good thing, but only for so long. Over and over, they were able to reroute with each breakdown, enabling them to maintain performance despite the continual overload. This is successful only up to a point. After a certain point, rerouting becomes inefficient and their overloaded system comes to a standstill. Even though they pushed to the point of tissue breakdown, we were able to regain function by removing each imbalance layer by layer. Their body needed a complete reboot and we were able to go through and reset all the breakers.

It took a few weeks of intensive work, but the dysfunctional pain and movement patterns that developed after many years of training returned back to normal. Our Olympic athlete was back on track and making plans to train for another world championship and Olympic team. They were able to increase the training load to their previous volume and add in the more intense workouts necessary to compete at that level. All this was done by letting the body communicate its built-in ability to heal.

As for our MS patient, when she initially came in, she had lost strength in her legs and was losing her ability to walk. Her doctors warned that her symptoms could progressively get worse or at best remain the same. Doctors told her she couldn't have any more children and she may need assistance in caring for her current children if the disease continued to progress. After a few months of treatment, which included dietary changes, targeted nutritional support, along with the treatment outlined above. She had regained full strength in her legs. The burning and tingling in her legs disappeared and she was able to care for her children. Fast-forward a few years, and she was surprised to add two more children to her family and an MRI showed her MS was in remission. The body has an amazing ability to repair when the barriers to healing are removed and proper communication is restored.

As we've outlined above, there are a number of built-in healing pathways that can be used to restore health. Our brain has an endless capacity for learning and healing, but unfortunately our information pathways can get bogged down from chronic levels of physical, chemical, and emotional stress, causing a breakdown in communication. By assisting our brain and body to process and remove these stressors with the techniques described in this chapter and in this book, health can be bountiful and our body's ability to heal can be lifted to levels that are truly remarkable.

About the Author

Dr. Noah J Moos

Dr. Noah Moos is a cum laude graduate from Logan Chiropractic College. Before attending chiropractic college, Dr. Moos was a collegiate track and field athlete where he competed at the National Championships in both cross-country and track and field. Dr. Moos is a thought leader and innovator in the area of alternative and complementary medicine. He is also the product developer for The Human Nutrition Project. Dr. Moos works with Olympic and professional athletes from different sports along with people who are considered medical mysteries or failures and everyone else in between.

He has a unique perspective on health, combining cutting-edge techniques with traditional wisdom. He has contributed internationally to events such as The International Symposium of Integrative Medicine in Beijing and has presented his unique concepts throughout the US. Dr. Moos is passionate about helping people get to the root cause of their condition and optimize their human potential.

Contact Information:
Health-Plus ATX
Website: www.healthplusaustin.com
Facebook: dr.noahmoos
Instagram: dr.noahmoos
Twitter: drnoahmoos

HEMP HEALING FOR A HAPPY HIPPOCAMPUS

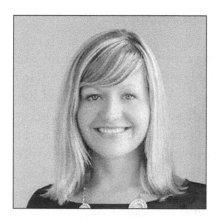

Dr. Puja Wentworth-Peters

The Fall

I don't recall whether I lost my balance or was pushed by the other kids head-first into the deep end of the empty swimming pool that day in 1982. I do recall witnessing the event from about 40 feet above my body. Looking down at my mother holding me, and at times rocking me back and forth as her tears fell upon my cheeks, I felt the distinct tug back and forth between the Earth below and the heavens above.

My mother tells me that my blue body felt like "Jello," and that the top of my skull resembled "Frito Pie." Her story also recounts that I would scream and then become completely quiet, but present.

I remember floating above, then dashing into my body with the perspective of her grieving face above me and feeling the immense pain. I would quickly dash above the two of us and remain perfectly quiet as if the unbearable pain had caused my soul to separate from my body.

I later learned that this was called an NDE (Near Death Experience), and that I had what is referred to as an "out of body experience," where the soul of a person is disconnected from their physical form through extreme trauma—literal disassociation. Thousands of individuals have reported similar experiences, and for me, this was the first of three.

Pain Will Live Here No More

The following morning I spoke to my shocked mother and said that "God had spoken to me." I said, "He had written on my brain with a silver pencil that pain would live here no more." It was not by coincidence or accident that I became fascinated with resilience and the power to bounce back and recover despite the odds. Ernest Hemingway once wrote, "The world breaks everyone and afterwards, many are strong at the broken places." These have been guiding words for me through the traumas and tragedies I have endured and flourished despite. In my experience, it is NOT a coincidence that some people become triumphant over their trauma, growing from pain to purpose. So, what are the recipes to this victory? First let me tell you about how one culture relishes the beauty of imperfection and suffering.

Kinsugi

In my personal and professional study of resilience and human potential, I often think of the Japanese practice of "Kinsugi," translated to "golden joinery." Kintsugi (or Kintsukuroi, which means "golden repair"), is the centuries-old Japanese art of fixing broken pottery with a special lacquer dusted with powdered gold, silver, or platinum. Beautiful seams of gold fill in the cracks of ceramic ware, giving a unique appearance to the piece. This repair method celebrates each artifact's unique history by emphasizing its fractures and breaks instead of hiding or disguising them. Kintsugi often makes the repaired piece even more beautiful than the original, revitalizing it with new life.

In the realm of trauma and post-traumatic stress, when

"Kinsugi" is applied to the human psyche, we find a level of healing and trauma recovery felt within the brain when the tragedy is no longer hidden, and the gifts of the pain are felt and understood. People who have endured the struggle, picked up the pieces and marched on again with grace, create hope for others who suffer.

I remember in 2013 upon realizing I had Lyme disease, how my heart dropped into the pit of my stomach followed by a chuckle—an ironic giggle. I thought to myself, "Well, thank you God. You know I am a kinesthetic learner, so therefore you have allowed me the opportunity to experience a traumatic birth, multiple car accidents, multiple traumatic brain injuries, amputation, autoimmune disease, severe anemia, spider bite paralysis from a black widow, face paralysis from a scorpion bite, divorce, mold exposure, mercury toxicity, and now Lyme."

I knew I would conquer and manage the consequences of such a painful "gift," for failure has never been an option for me—just learnings. I knew that somehow the great learning I would experience firsthand would be worth the pain, although sometimes it seemed too unbearable. Letting the "golden joinery" occur in my own life prepared me for the empathy needed for the other "perfectly imperfect" souls I would meet in my wellness clinics and retreats.

Out-of-Control Stress

You see, I was off-balance that day next to the pool because I was still recovering from an unfortunate motorcycle accident that had occurred a few months prior, where my left foot was amputated. The five or so pints of blood loss left me needing a blood transfusion in 1981. I later worried so much about the possible tainted blood supply of that time period that I was tested for AIDS every six months for five years.

With this amount of trauma, it's no surprise that I was then diagnosed with juvenile rheumatoid arthritis at the age of eight. In my experience as a health practitioner who has helped many chronically ill individuals, there is always an immense history of stress and trauma preceding an autoimmune reaction. This stress level is different for everyone, and the consequence is based on that person's capacity for resilience to stress.

The stress we endure has its consequences such as overwhelm, depression, insomnia, body pain, weight loss resistance, increased heart disease, cancer and dementia/Alzheimer's have become the norm. The physiologic stress response produces one of the most lifesaving in the short term, and life devastating substances in the long term. I consider adrenaline and cortisol to be two of the most toxic substances to the human body. Yes, over the long term, elevated cortisol levels can be as detrimental to overall health as excessive blood sugar is for diabetes or Alzheimer's (now termed Type III diabetes). Stress profoundly injures your brain.

Elevated cortisol levels make you weight loss resistant, kill your sex drive, shrink your brain, compromise your immune system, and generally make you feel terrible. Besides the tendencies towards anxiety and depression, many people begin carrying extra adipose tissue around their belly. This type of fat is also highly associated with the development of the top three killers: heart disease, diabetes, and cancer.

Elevated cortisol levels resulting from chronic stress have also been associated with decreased muscle mass, decreased bone density, memory and learning impairment, increased symptoms of PMS, cramps, increased or decreased appetite, and increased menopausal side effects like hot flashes and night sweats.

Stressed-out

The difference between stress and being stressed out is that being stressed induces adaptive responses in which the hormone cortisol goes up and then comes down quickly, whereas being stressed out suggests an inability to regulate the body's stress response. Salivary or urine cortisol testing tells us that the cortisol rhythm stays flat so that overall cortisol exposure over 24 hours is actually higher than if it spiked early and then came down within a 24-hour period.

In fact, it is this non-adaptive course of systemic events that many believe leads to most of the common diseases of modern life. Dutch neurology researchers have also observed the same patterns of flattened cortisol rhythm and non-adaptive stress response in chronic fatigue, fibromyalgia, PTSD, depression, and burn out. These detrimental stress cascades lead to the shrinking of a particular part of the brain called the hippocampus.

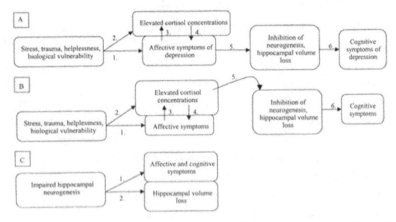

Proc Natl Acad Sci U.S.A. Depression, antidepressants, and the shrinking hippocampus (2001).

Trauma Hijacking

Have you ever felt hijacked by your emotions? Yes, our brains are wired for memory and even more so, negative experience memories called negative bias. When the memory is disturbed and involves cortisol and other stress responses, the brain remembers the incident in even more vivid color.

I remember precisely the most distinct details from the day of the motorcycle accident. I remember I was so proud of my new brown, brushed leather school shoes and the purple knee-high socks I chose to wear that morning of the accident. I remember the flashing of the lights on the motorcycle as the engine stalled once my foot had jammed the rotation of the chain.

I remember pulling my foot out of the grips of the biting chain. I remember the bearded man in a maroon Buick (I think), my angel, the angel from nowhere who took my dad and I to the hospital in Lewistown, Montana that November evening. I remember being triaged quickly and then sent in an ambulance for a very long ride miles away to Billings, Montana where I had emergency surgery and a blood transfusion. I remember all the letters that my kindergarten classmates sent to me and I remember crawling up and down the stairs of my attic bedroom. I remember learning how to walk again, stepping from square to square of my parent's Afghan rug they brought back from the motorcycle journey around the world.

What we know through neuroscience now is that with significant trauma, the memories connected to the stress of the incident hijack your frontal cortex from rational thought, and all that is left is fear and reactivity. The part of your brain most responsible for memory and fear responses is the hippocampus. People who experience chronic "post-traumatic stress response" to simple life stressors develop decreased hippocampal size. (8) When our brain has been affected by chronic, ongoing stress, cortisol enters the body and causes a cascade of inflammatory effects, incredibly damaging to the body as I have said previously. As cortisol increases, insulin increases, and pro-inflammatory cytokines begin a cascade of pain-inducing inflammatory responses that further injure internal organs and brain cells.

The Hippocampus

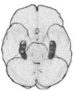

Henceforth, here enters the topic of the lesser known part of the brain known as "the hippocampus," meaning "sea horse," because of its c-curved shape intimately entwined with the amygdala, the emotional center of our brain. The hippocampus is one of the most vital and fascinating parts of the brain. Located under the cerebral cortex, it is a central component of the limbic system, the emotional center of the brain, and is responsible for forming, consolidating, and storing memories, emotional learning and regulation, decision-making, creativity, empathy, and spatial orientation.

Hippocampus abnormalities are implicated in a range of cognitive and emotional disorders, including Alzheimer's disease, schizophrenia, and transient global amnesia. Researchers have found that traumatic events and severe stress can cause shrinkage of this area of the brain, with significant changes observed in both men and women who suffer from post-traumatic stress disorder, especially as the result of sexual assault or combat.

Hippocampus Shrinkage and Depression

Are you wondering if this could be you? In the case of depression for example, atrophy of the hippocampus impairs the ability to experience a healthy range of emotions and to regulate those emotions in a normal way. You may be less able to control your impulses and adapt to change while becoming predisposed to negative thought patterns that are difficult to break out of. You may be more likely to engage in self-destructive activity, including substance abuse. Hippocampal shrinkage also damages cognitive functions and interferes with the process of creating memories, which has a profound impact on both behavior and the ability to form a stable, realistic, and cohesive sense of self. Memory dysregulation can be a key factor in depressive experiences and closely affect both emotional states and your overall identity. Hippocampal changes also interfere with your ability to form and maintain healthy social relationships and make good social decisions.

A 2014 study in the *Journal of Frontiers in Human Neuroscience* in fact found that damage to the hippocampus can hinder flexible cognitive and social behavior by preventing you from accurately interpreting and responding to information. (1) Social bonding is impaired, as is accurate judgment of character, and even your ability to use language effectively. Over the years, as I personally experienced the majority of these consequences, I sought out every avenue of healing that made sense to me and a few that did not. In the end, it was legal cannabis (7) that changed the tide and dropped my levels of inflammation so drastically in my brain and body that I could continue to care for others that, to me, seemed in worse need.

Hemp, Hemp Hooray!

In 2013, when I realized I had Lyme disease, triggered by a home with mold in the walls, I leaned in heavily to the anti-inflammatory power of cannabinoids (with less than .3% THC) to successfully allow me the ability to continue working in my busy wellness practice. Cannabinoids have such a profound effect on regulating the body through their activation of our endocannabinoid system (ECS) that many consider them to be a "Panacea from the Heavens."

The ECS is the number one regulator of the entire neurotransmitter system. It has actually been recognized as an important modulator in the function of brain, endocrine, and immune tissues. It also has been recognized through research as the regulatory role in the secretion of hormones related to reproductive functions and responses to stress.

Although this system is found in all mammals, in humans it controls energy balance, food intake centers of the central nervous system, and gastrointestinal tract activity. "The endocannabinoid system regulates not only the central and peripheral mechanisms of food intake, but also lipids synthesis and turnover in the liver and adipose tissue as well as glucose metabolism in muscle cells." (2)

It was not until recent years that this ECS (endocannabinoid system) master regulating system of the whole body began being taught in medical schools. In fact, in 2013 only a mere 13% of medical schools even mentioned the ECS. The forefront of cannabis research has been done by Professor Raphael Mechoulam, a scientist at the Hebrew University in Israel. Mechoulam, the leading pioneer in this field of understanding, was the first to isolate, analyze and synthesize the major psychoactive and non-psychoactive compounds in cannabis and has developed a number of revolutionary cannabis-related treatments. It is known that endocannabinoids are effective in lowering inflammation and providing antioxidant capabilities to the body, thus being a "rescue receptor" that upregulates in times of trouble. Several studies also suggest that these cannabinoids inhibit cancer growth by inducing cell death in tumor cells.

Today, roughly 147 million people use cannabis for effective relief of their troubles. I am always interested in the wisdom we once knew. For me, learning that 90% of the medicine between 1850 and 1936 was cannabis-derived and lead by the pharmaceutical industry, especially Eli Lilly, further fueled my belief that hemp was a key component to a happy brain.

The THC Hippocampal Shrinkage Issue

When I speak of cannabis, I speak of low THC versions. In the United States, anything with less than .3% THC is what is now considered federally legal. I had heard for years that cannabis was medicine, but it took a while to discern the differences. In recent years, scientists have determined that the THC caused focalized shrinking of hippocampus volume. Now in a recent 2018 Cannabis and Cannabinoid Research article (3), this negative outcome with chronic cannabis use is further associating with neuroanatomical alterations in the hippocampus.

These researchers reported, "While adverse impacts of cannabis use are generally attributed to Δ9-tetrahydrocannabinol (THC), emerging naturalistic evidence suggests cannabidiol (CBD) is neuroprotective and may ameliorate brain harms associated with cannabis use, including protection from hippocampal volume loss. This study examined whether prolonged administration of CBD to regular cannabis users within the community could reverse or reduce the characteristic hippocampal harms associated with chronic Cannabis use."(4)

While I believe there are synergistic effects that can take place with the inclusion of very low THC known to many as the "entourage effect," in the 1970s the THC level in most cannabis was 7-8%; now, the levels are often 18-35% THC which when used chronically would further hippocampal shrinkage and potentially will exacerbate psychological dysfunction like dementia, Alzheimer's, schizophrenia and depression.(4)

The CBD Hippocampal Expansion

Science now teaches us that the cannabis component known as CBD (Cannabidiol) which is one of over a hundred cannabinoids of the Cannabis plant, is indeed neuroprotective and in fact, the National Institute of Health holds a patent on this fact. CBD has even been connected to the brain recovery of chronic THC users who have experienced the shrinkage of their hippocampus from THC use.

My greatest interest regarding trauma memories was the new understanding that the activation of the CB1 receptors in particular in the brain assisted in the mind's recovery of negative memories. This means that with the proper usage of cannabinoids, adverse memories that hijack the hippocampus and therefore a person's emotions and happy brain, are being discovered to dissolve in their fear responses, leaving only a mild existence of their presence.

Brain Resilience

It was not by coincidence or accident that I became fascinated with resilience and the power to bounce back and recover despite the odds. There are many ways to heal a saddened brain, but these are a few of my most important ones in my own personal victory:

- *Have an "attitude of gratitude" even for the small blessings*
- *Focus on 7.5-9 hours of sleep per night.*
- *Hydrate with electrolyte-filled reverse osmosis water (half your body weight in ounces and more if you exercise daily).*
- *Correct the electro-smog within your home and work environment.*
- *Find a healing modality that works for you (i.e., chiropractic, acupuncture, massage).*
- *Release the "issues from your tissues" by finding a Body Code Practitioner.*
- *Incorporate daily photobiomodulation (PBM) into your life.* The power of this brain and body modality to dissolve amyloid plaque is reason enough.
- *Take a Daily DHA Supplement* – DHA or Docosahexaenoic acid is an Omega-3 that is a central building block of brain tissue. DHA is thought to combat the inflammatory effects of cortisol and the plaque buildup associated with vulnerability to Alzheimer's disease. "According to Dr. Mehmet Oz, in one study, a dose of 600mg of DHA taken daily for 6 months led the brain to perform as if it were three years younger." Incorporating omega-3 fatty acids overall allows for

greater activation of the endocannabinoid system with the use of cannabinoids.

- ***Activate your endocannabinoid system with organic cannabinoids containing low THC and high CBD.*** Start low and slow at about 25mg each day and double the dose until you find a dose that makes you feel more happy, healthy, and whole. There is value in incorporating various cannabinoids. Once you find this personalized dose that is different for everyone, continue at this dose for four months and then begin to lower dosage to a satisfactory maintenance dose for daily consumption.

My personal story began with 30mg per day in 2013 to assist my Lyme symptoms to later realizing its other profound effects regarding hippocampal healing and happiness lead me to four months of 400mg per day. I have even read stories of medical doctors treating their patients with brain tumors with a three-month protocol of 1000mg/day. (6)

Vagus Nerve Activation and a Happy Hippocampus

There are two parts of the nervous system that control our daily functioning. The "fight or flight system" is the sympathetic nervous system and the "stay and play" or "rest and digest" system is the parasympathetic nervous system. The vagus nerve is the tenth cranial nerve and controls the parasympathetic side of our nervous system that controls the functioning of our entire existence. It extends from its origin in the brainstem through the neck and the thorax down to the abdomen.

Because of its long path through the human body, it has also been described as the "wanderer nerve." In the neck, the vagus nerve provides required innervation to most of the muscles that control breathing, swallowing, eating, speaking, digesting and facial expression. It provides the main parasympathetic supply to the heart, and in fact stimulates a reduction in our heart rate.

The brain–gut axis is becoming increasingly important as a therapeutic target for gastrointestinal and psychiatric disorders, such as inflammatory bowel disease, depression, and post-traumatic stress disorder. The gut is an important control center of the immune system and the vagus nerve is an immune system modulator. As a result, this nerve plays an important role in the relationship between the gut, the brain, and inflammation. Endocannabinoids (those our body naturally makes) are one of the main systems controlling both excitatory and inhibitory neurotransmission, as well as neuroplasticity within the hippocampus and activation of the vagus nerve, and therefore, the parasympathetic nervous system. Thus, by activating our endocannabinoid system, we drastically increase our body's ability to focus on repair by activating the vagus nerve. (5)

Happy Hippocampus, Happy You!

Let's learn from the art of Kinsugi. Similar to filling your broken places with gold to increase the beauty and functioning of your vessel, I would propose that we fill our receptors up with cannabinoids, assisting our precious hippocampus in lowering our fear responses, allowing our body the ability to drop our cytokines and other inflammatory markers, and therefore let us live happier lives. In addition to adding regular exercise to our weekly regimen, taking new routes on our drive home, and sharing new experiences which all excite hippocampal activity, incorporating high-quality cannabinoids is one of the best ways to increase our brain resilience.

Since we can't always control how much we are exposed to financial, relationship, illness, or trauma stress, let's revel in the preventive activities we can do to maintain cognitive resilience so we can continue to deal effectively with the stressors in our lives. As we activate our endocannabinoid system's CB1 and CB2 receptors, we become "antifragile" increasing our capacity to what life throws at us. In the realm of trauma and post-traumatic stress, when Kinsugi is applied to humanity, we find that beauty is found in our imperfections. We become forever resilient.

Citations:

(1) Front. Hum. Neurosci., 30 September 2014 | https://doi.org/10.3389/fnhum.2014.00742. **The role of the hippocampus in flexible cognition and social behavior.** Rachael D. Rubin,

Patrick D. Watson, Melissa C. Duff and Neal J. Cohen

(2) Postepy Hig Med Dosw (Online). 2007;61:99-105. [The role of the endocannabinoid system in the regulation of endocrine function and in the control of energy balance in humans]. [Article in Polish] Komorowski J1, Stepień H.

(3) Cannabis Cannabinoid Res. 2018; 3(1): 94–107. Published online 2018 Apr 1. doi: 10.1089/can.2017.0047 PMCID: PMC5908414 PMID: 29682609 **Prolonged Cannabidiol Treatment Effects on Hippocampal Subfield Volumes in Current Cannabis Users,** Camilla Beale, Samantha J. Broyd, Yann Chye, Chao Suo, Mark Schira, Peter Galettis, Jennifer H. Martin, Murat Yücel, and Nadia Solowij.

(4) Cannabis Cannabinoid Res. 2018; 3(1): 94–107. Published online 2018 Apr 1. doi: 10.1089/can.2017.0047 PMCID: PMC5908414 PMID: 29682609 **Prolonged Cannabidiol Treatment Effects on Hippocampal Subfield Volumes in Current Cannabis Users,** Camilla Beale, Samantha J. Broyd, Yann Chye, Chao Suo, Mark Schira, Peter Galettis, Jennifer H. Martin, Murat Yücel, and Nadia Solowij.

(5) Front Psychiatry. 2018 Mar 13;9:44. doi: 10.3389/fpsyt.2018.00044. eCollection 2018. **Vagus Nerve as Modulator of the Brain-Gut Axis in Psychiatric and Inflammatory Disorders.** Breit S, Kupferberg A, Rogler G, Hasler G.

(6) Br J Clin Pharmacol. 2013 Feb; 75(2): 303–312. Published online 2012 Apr 17. doi: 10.1111/j.1365-2125.2012.04298.x PMCID: PMC3579246 PMID: 22506672, **Cannabidiol as Potential Anticancer Drug,** Paola Massi, Marta Solinas, Valentina Cinquina, and Daniela Parolaro

(7) Front Behav Neurosci. 2013; 7: 124. Published online 2013 Sep 19. doi: 10.3389/fnbeh.2013.00124 PMCID: PMC3776936 PMID: 24065899, **Targeting the Endocannabinoid System to Treat Haunting Traumatic Memories,** Irit Akirav

(8) Dialogues Clin Neurosci. 2006 Dec; 8(4): 445–461. PMCID: PMC3181836 PMID: 17290802 **Traumatic Stress: Effects on the Brain,** J. Douglas Bremner, MD

About the Author

Dr. Puja Wentworth-Peters, DC

The Hemp Doctor and Inflammation Whisperer

Dr. Puja has been improving the cellular resilience of her clients since 2003 and in private practice in central North Carolina and working virtually since 2007. She is a Doctor of Chiropractic, functional wellness practitioner and human potential educator of epigenetic resilience, helping people heal their brain and nervous system naturally.

She believes "healing truly comes from "above down, inside out," for we are "self-healing, self-regulating organisms" designed to gain balance with proper nutrition, harmonizing and removal of interferences. Using training in chiropractic, functional medicine, nutrigenomics, neurofeedback, biofeedback, light and sound frequency therapy, nutrition, and cellular detoxification, she supports people getting their lives back so they can live their God-given potential.

Contact Information:
Website: www.wellcenteredwellness.com
Facebook: www.facebook.com/puja.wentworth,
          www.facebook.com/wellcenteredwellness/
Instagram: www.instagram.com/dr_puja/
          www.instagram.com/frequencylabapex/
LinkedIn: www.linkedin.com/pujawentworthdc

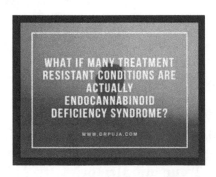

OBSERVATION IS THE ONLY KEY FOR TRANSFORMATION:
Awareness will lead to salvation and FREEDOM to be!

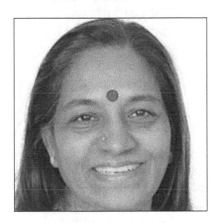

Dr. Rita Mahajan

Let me admit at the outset that I write this article as a person who is inspired by many of the scientists I have been following, read, and understand. I was offered the opportunity to write this book along with those I had always admired to the likes of Dr. Bruce Lipton, who had inspired me with his work, Dr. Paul Drouin, founder of Quantum University and who has brought together people from various continents and offering a unique education, Dr. Patrick Porter, who has brought in so many simple tools with his visualization guided meditations with light and sound for anyone to use, Dr. Amit Goswami, and others.

Simplicity is their strength; so is mine.

There are many masters in every stage of my life, and I had

the good fortune of meeting and learning from them. I have lived my life with intuition that guided me perfectly. Looking back, I feel overwhelmed with the divine plan like puzzle pieces coming together to form a picture. It gives me great strength in knowing that I am always guided, and it leaves me freer to flow with life. It is my honour to be a part of this new book called *Wake UP: The Happy Brain.*

In this new age, we need tools for our everyday (healthy) living. Simple tools, simple understanding, and simple application. Spiritual science and its application for everyday healthy living this is what I call my work. Anyone can access the power of healthy living with observation and awareness. I am writing my perspective of these matters without any prejudice to anyone living or otherwise. It is purely my thoughts and I have found power in these approaches, so I hope you will be able to access the same.

While we have the abilities to understand, comprehend, and apply the principles of life, it begins with observation—observing things AS THEY ARE; only then we can be aware of them. This will give us access to awareness of our perspectives that leads to our actions/reactions. If we continue to do this regularly, this will become our FIXED WAY of operations on a daily basis. Observation is the ability to be neutral, without judgement, without prejudice, and taking our ego away from the equation.

Awareness is the ability to feel, perceive, know, and be conscious of our existence. All things in the Universe have awareness but in different levels. As human beings, we have expanded our awareness to the level of self-awareness. This is the level of awareness that separates us from rocks, plants, and animals. Having the ability of self-awareness can be a blessing, but it can also be a curse.

Self-awareness allows us to sense that we are separated from each other. It will lead us to realise we are unique, and this can boost our egos more. If we are led to understand that we are in essence the same but in different forms, constitutions, colour, and creed, it will lead to experience oneness. In truth, there is no separation because we are all connected and made of the same substances. Having the ability to feel separated from each other and Creation (God) gives us the illusion of more freedom and makes life more interesting. It allows us to explore reality in our own ways through the use of free will. Externalizing God

(Creation) as separate from us gives us a sense of God out there. The awareness of self is the one other form of manifestation of "that which is" can give us more sense of oneness!

Having a strong self-awareness is one of our greatest protections against negative forces. Most people do not understand how powerful their awareness is. Our awareness can be our access to salvation. Through knowledge of self-empowerment and learning life lessons, we can expand our awareness to a state of pure cognition, a state of all knowing. At this state we cannot be deceived or manipulated, because we will know when someone is trying to harm or lie to us.

When we observe and become aware, we can distinguish past, present, and future events. We can change our thought patterns toward what we want, which will change what manifests into our reality. Because our consciousness is still in a baby-like state, changes may not seem significant because of the way our awareness processes time. If we lose focus of our desires before they manifest, we will deny ourselves those desires. If we can find a likeminded group to help focus their thought patterns to what we are focusing on, we can speed up the manifestation process. The more people, the better results.

Being more aware can help us expand our consciousness. As our consciousness expands, it increases our energy frequency. Once we reach a certain level of frequency, we can become immune to the influence of negative forces and diseases. We can stand in nothing 24/7, 365 days and flow with life. As we are more available to life, our frequencies attract those things that need attention. By giving our attention, we create. We not only impact or own lives and everyone around us. It is another level of peeling the onion and revealing another level of creation. More gratitude, less conflict. What else can you ask for? Perfection in the way it is is the game.

"Enlightenment is every day in the NOW moment.
Yesterday's enlightenment is today's ego trip."

Creating a Healthy Planet with Healthy Human Beings

We can live a healthy life. Having said that about health, I have observed that the potential of business in the medical and wellness industries have doubled and tripled over last two decades. There are more and more advanced technologies that deal with complicated medical conditions. Our country is known for Ayurveda and natural medicine, yet there are more than enough hospitals and wellness clinics and but no solutions. There are more people in hospitals than in shopping malls. This observation leads me to think where we are heading, and which direction humanity is going.

At one end of the pendulum, we are advancing in our understanding of self and the Universe, and information technology has entered almost every area of life. On the other end, we find more pollution and more people seeking medical help. This was reinforced by a statistical report I read in 2014. The world-famous analyst had come up with a figure of potential business of $450 Billion in the wellness industry in 2012 and predicted it to be $960 Billion by 2015. I was shocked. It led me to wonder if we are doubling the number of sick people or that of potential business. Potential growth means potential seekers of health care. It means greater numbers of people are falling ill. Once a person falls ill, we compromise harmony, lifestyle, and money.

I began to ponder over the fact and waited for 2015 to see what we had achieved. Alarmingly, we reached $1,500 Billion and overshot the expected predictions of the potential wellness industry's growth. In 2020, the predicted amount is estimated to be $150,000 Billion. This left me baffled, so I took a break and started reconsidering my life. At the end of my observation and awareness, I took the first step forward and started a Center for Quantum Energy Medicine and began to propagate a new paradigm for healthcare.

In my own little way, I began to deliver lectures wherever possible and started planting a seed of hope that we must be responsible for the only home we live in called EARTH. This is the only PLANET OF CHOICE, and therefore as the inhabitants of this planet, we must be responsible for the wellbeing of ourselves first, thereby contributing to the energy of the Earth field. If we are healthy, we contribute to the energy field of our environment, thereby creating a coherence of a harmonious energy around us.

How do we expand our awareness? Begin with observing every thought you have. How often do you repeat the same thoughts? Is the thought in the affirmative, positive, or negative? This will lead you to understand your own thought patterns. Most of us are used to only thinking the opposite of our intention. We are not precise in our thoughts. They are random and mostly based on our negative past experiences. For example, we will want to go ahead and be successful, yet our thoughts will be, "I do not want to fail." If you observe and bring to awareness that you are thinking exactly to the opposite of your intention, then you can change it to reflect your intention and not the other way around.

Listed below are some ways you can achieve this:

- **Increase self-empowerment:** As you increase your self-empowerment, you strengthen your connection to other beings because you are becoming less fearful of others and the unknown. Once you see yourself in others, it leaves you freer to be yourself.

- **Be aware of your fear:** Fear is what prevents you from expanding your awareness because it puts you in a state of denial. It will also make you feel isolated from the world. In a way, you will live in a separatist concept and therefore you fear that others are out to get you. If you begin to observe that all around you are your own manifestations in different forms, you will feel at home and it will empower you.

- **Reduce self-pity "distraction":** Self-pity is a powerful distraction from SELF! Distraction reduces or blocks the connection to your inner awareness. This blockage suppresses your mind and prevents it from expanding its awareness. Distraction also prevents you from contemplating your thoughts, further preventing you from knowing who you truly are. You cannot expand your awareness unless you understand who you are.

- **Thoughts create:** The fact that you have thoughts should be good enough proof that you are a being with infinite potential. Thought is one of the most powerful energy forces in the Universe. It is one of the fundamental forces of Creation because it is needed to focus everything into existence.

- **Overcome denial:** Being in a state of denial prevents you from accessing higher levels of consciousness, because it sets a parameter around your awareness and locks you in. As long as you are locked in this box of denial, you will have a very hard time expanding your awareness. To rise above this box, you will need to face your fears, be open-minded, and think outside of the box.

- **Strengthen your intuition:** Your intuition is another part of your awareness. It is a knowingness that takes place at the cellular levels. Some of us like to refer to it as a "gut feeling." To strengthen your intuition, you will need to observe when the quiet whisper, gut feeling, or small voice is prompting you. This will lead to understanding inner guidance and I promise you, you can never go wrong. This is because our intuition is a default program which is built within each one of us as a guiding factor. You cannot afford to ignore this. You will need to learn how to discern your intelligent thoughts given by your past experiences to that of the inner voice. It will enable you to access higher levels of your consciousness. This can be accomplished through meditation and DNA activation.

- **Reduce the power of your ego:** This is easier said than done. Even today, we still do not fully understand the EGO. We think it is something very bad. I think it is the self that you know and understand in its fullest potential of what is possible and your limitations. It is the one that you are comfortable with and you think is truly YOU!

  Your ego/identity is another part of your awareness that you know and understand. It has been isolated from your intuition, subconscious, conscious, and higher self. It is an awareness that is lost, desperate, and confused. Its main goal is survival. Because of the way it sees itself and thinks, it tries to put you in a state of denial so it can overpower you. This prevents your awareness from expanding. To reduce the power of your ego, you will need to take personal responsibility for your actions, so do not give away your powers to your ego. The ego is a part of who you are; fearing it will only strengthen its power. Instead of fearing it, you should work with it to bring it back into balance. I call this a personality that is in FIXED operative mode. Once you observe your thoughts and action/reaction, you will be led to be aware that it is limited and does not enable you to go beyond the limit it has set forth. You will need to break this limitation. You just can't break it unless you have brought it to your awareness by keenly observing it. Only then you have access to be or do differently. This way, it will lead you to explore beyond the limitation.

- **Increase your energy frequency:** The world beyond matter is built on energy. Frequency is the code that gives energy expression. In order to expand your awareness, you will need to increase your energy frequency. Doing this will allow you to access higher levels of consciousness; therefore, expanding your awareness beyond your wildest dreams. Healing your light body and DNA and meditating on a regular basis are three effective techniques for increasing your energy frequency. There are other effective methods, like letting go and laughing at your own follies and being with people without judgement or opinions. This is being in a state of freedom to be.

- **Most importantly standing for who you are!** You are a DIVINE being in the Human form. You can call it by the name of GOD or anything else. I call it "THAT WHICH IS." Remembering this on an everyday basis will enable you to be manifesting all that you need to fulfil your daily life. It will give a great grounding and to stand for yourself. It will no longer be a SURVIVAL of the fittest. Survival of the fittest creates conflict, not cooperation and coexistence. When you stand for who you are as the DIVINE BEING IN HUMAN MANIFESTATION, you can live in coexistence create harmony.

- **Write your own script and moving forward in life.** As you live your life on an everyday basis, one day at a time, you write your own history. Looking back, you feel proud of those moments of failures, moments of humiliation, conflicts, and disappointments that have led to the refined, self-empowered being that you are today.

- **My greatest advice:** Human existence is the most beautiful of all the other existences. In this form what you think, what you do, and what you feel impacts not only your own body, but others around you, your family, the environment, the planet, as well as the Universe. **Therefore, by having the power of observation and bringing to awareness, you can make a huge difference in writing the script of our future world.** How would you want to see this planet in the next 500 years? What kind of an education you would like to impart today that future generations will be able to take forward for the next emerging galactic human?

- **What kind of resources would you like to leave that will enable the Earth's transformation, meaning the transformation of Earthlings?** Can we create a heaven on earth today, thereby leaving a legacy of a healthy planet? It is no longer rocket science. We all can start with ourselves and contribute to the collective coherence of our planet.

I love you all! Be safe, observe, be aware, and be in action. Play the game of life full-throttle as of right now. This is one lifetime, and we all can make a huge difference!

About the Author

Dr. Rita Mahajan

A CHANNEL FOR THE DIVINE to express itself.

Dr. Mahajan has a PhD in quantum energy medicine from the International University for Complementary and Alternative Medicine. She is the Director of WOQEM Research Center.

Coming from a humble Army family and brought up as a Roman Catholic, she had a disciplined upbringing in a large joint family. Highly regarded for her pious and quiet nature and coming from a conservative family, she broke the rules by going to a co-education college and graduated with a degree in commerce. Her aspiration was to become a medical doctor. When she had the opportunity, she joined a diploma course in medical lab technology. She was always multitasking and learning all the time.

Rita never stopped her pursuit of medicine and jumped into the idea of starting a surgical instruments business in 1984. She established this business with a couple of industries, producing one of the finest surgical instruments in the country.

In 2011 and given by her strong inner call, Dr. Mahajan began to diversify in the field of spiritual science and had started to give workshops all over India on cosmic ray activation, DNA activation, auras, and chakras. She has organised many conferences: 1st World Parliament on Spirituality, WOQEM 2016, 2017, 2018 and many others.

She has now integrated all that she does under World of Quantum Energy Medicine and delivers lectures all over the world. She has been recognised by many organisations and been awarded, with one of the most prestigious awards being the Mahatma Gandhi Leadership Award 2019 in the House of Commons, London and the Women in Leadership Award 2016 by ISBR Management School. She has received many leadership awards from Lions Clubs International for her services.

Contact Information:
Quantum Energy Medicine
Tel: +919739076535 / +91 080 41313777
Websites: www.woqem.com
            www.mahajanophthalmic.in
            www.divinelearningunlimited.com
            www.consciousparentingresearchfoundation.org
Email: info@woqem.com

UNLOCKING THE NEUROLOGICAL CODE FOR HEATH, WEALTH, VITALITY, AND OPTIMAL HUMAN PERFORMANCE

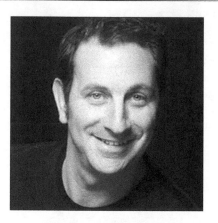

Dr. Steven Schwartz

What if I told you there is a very specific code that is contained within our nervous system, that, when activated, unlocks and reveals the secrets to obtaining optimal health, wealth, vitality and optimal human performance? This notion may sound like something right out of a science fiction movie, however, the information I am about to share with you is rooted in established scientific fact and is easily accessible simply by understanding key components.

The nervous system is a complex system that consists of many different components, most commonly, the brain and spinal cord, which make up the central nervous system (CNS). The nerves that extend from the spine and supply energy to every tissue, system, and cell of the body is called the peripheral nervous system (PNS). These two subdivisions of the nervous system are simply no more than relay stations to receive, process, interpret, and express information from our environment. There is another primary neurological system that I refer to as the "true" nervous system and is the most direct access point into the other two systems, known as the connective tissue matrix (CTM).

By definition, the connective tissue matrix, explained by Dr. James Oschman in his book, *The Scientific Basis of Energy Medicine*, refers to the living connective tissue matrix as an underlying material of the body that connects all of our tissues together.

As stated in my book, *Primal Resonance, Discover the Secrets to Health, Vitality and Optimal Human Performance,* "The language of the cell is that of vibrational resonance."

There is a specific anatomical framework that connects your cells and all of your physiology together. This framework is what allows your cells to communicate easily, effortlessly, constantly, and continuously throughout your lifetime. It is a brilliant system, created for efficiency. The efficiency of this system is actually responsible for chronic disease being so widespread in our modern world because cellular communication continually does what it was trained to do over time; it remembers and perpetuates patterns.

There are three primary biological materials that make up the living connective tissue matrix: microfilaments, microtubules, and intermediate tubules. Their function is to interact with and interpret the external and internal environment through vibrational resonance. These vibrationally resonating materials reside in every tissue, system, and cell of the body and are the initiating materials with the process of mitosis, how our cells replicate, and signal transduction, how our cells communicate.

How does mitosis, signal transduction, the central nervous system, and living connective matrix have to do with health, wealth, and optimal human performance? The connective tissue feeds the brain and spinal cord, influencing the way our body releases chemicals.

If you are sad, angry, and self-deprecating, or happy, successful, and healthy, it is a neurological expression of

how your environment, past memories/associations and the nervous system interact with one another. This is a foundational principle to understand. The following codes are the core pillars for unlocking the highest potential of your neurological expression.

The Five Neurological Codes for Health, Wealth, and Optimal Human Performance:

1. Dimensional Shifting. We are physical manifestations of our own energetic expressions.
2. Causal Chain Progression. The key to reversing chronic illness, emotional distress, and overall dissidence in your body.
3. Cellular Memory. The missing link for human optimization.
4. Vibrational Resonance. The language of the body.
5. Water. The vital medium for cellular activation.

Dimensional Shifting: We Are Physical Manifestations of Our Own Energetic Expression

Whether you are a pro elite athlete, crippled with a debilitating disease, ultra-wealthy, or hopelessly broke, you are the physical expression of that energy. You are the physical manifestation of your own energetic expression. Understanding this concept and how to align into a new energetic expression of your choosing is known as dimensional shifting.

Step one, own all aspects of who you are. We have been shaped, molded, and refined over the years by our parents, romantic partners, business associates, and other life experiences, good and bad, that have created a unique individual expression of who we are.

In my practice, I would treat a significant number of patients going through a divorce. I used to say to them, "You may be legally divorced, but are you energetically divorced?" **How many experiences in your life are you still blaming others for or holding onto resentment for years after the initial trauma?**

You may be legally separated from that trauma. However, are you still energetically perpetuating that same trauma? Are you still the physical manifestation of that past trauma or are you aligned into a new reality? The "signaling" of your past experiences are anchored in your cells and that vibration is then left to be processed and interpreted by your brain and other components of your nervous system.

As we travel deeper inside our cells, we begin to see we are more empty potential energy than physical matter. We operate in the realm of the atom and its components of protons, neutrons and electrons. Protons and neutrons form the middle of the atom with electrons orbiting around the outside. All three vibrate, with the most movement occurring with electrons. As electrons move between areas called "shells" or "clouds," they release energy and activate a spark as they jump from shell to shell or move through clouds. This process is known as photonic emission. Light is given off every time an electron jumps to a different energy level.

In every cell in your body, there are countless numbers of atoms and even smaller more numerous electrons. This phenomenon ripples throughout every cell in your body. Imagine what that would look like, an infinite number of sparks produced from photonic emission. This is you. This bright light has been referred to as your biofield, your aura, or energy field. This compilation of light is your energetic expression. As you change the orientation of the electrons in the shells, you change the way you express yourself. **Change the way light expresses itself in your body and you change who you are.** Scientific research shows that laser and therapeutic light can successfully influence electron shell orientation.

Sound is light slowed down. Compare the speed of light to the speed of sound. Sound is much slower and is a shorter wavelength on the electromagnetic field spectrum. This is why you can see lightning before you hear thunder. This is why sound and vibration are such a fantastic delivery system for directly influencing neurology. Sound, light frequency, and vibration can literally change your entire biological expression and physical reality. With these tools and codes, you can ground and align into a new dimension of your choosing.

Dimensional shifting is a process of changing from one "measurable space" to another. Your current reality is one measurable space. How much money you make? Who are you in a relationship with? Where do you live? Are you happy? Are you sick? You are the physical expression of your electrons orienting to align in your current reality. What reality do you want to align with? Do you want to be healthier? Do you want to make more money? Do you want to be in a great loving respectful relationship? What dimensions have you not given yourself permission to activate?

Dimensional shifting is a practice of "disorganizing" your physical reality and changing the way your electrons orient themselves so that they are in alignment with any dimension of your choosing. For now, simply ponder the possibilities of spinning electrons coupled with your intention and the notion that you can reorganize into a new reality. You are the physical manifestation of your own energetic expression.

Causal Chain Progression

Every aspect of our modern culture is a byproduct of reactionary cause and effects symptomatic-based behavior. If we are sad, angry, frustrated, poor, sick or depressed, we reactionarily compensate with a variety of activities ranging from drugs, food, alcohol, sex, movies, exercise, and even career paths. The modern healthcare model is predominantly symptom-based care. You can google a common ailment and a variety of "remedies" that relieve symptoms will appear.

In the early days of my practice, I learned about fundamental "causes" that activates the immune system and nervous system into a hyperactive response. The most common categories are toxins and pathogens. These two very common triggers need to be corrected, balanced, reduced, and ideally eliminated from the body to produce long-term correction. There is another piece to the puzzle. Why are toxins and pathogens so predominant, and why do they not affect every person the same way?

In the early 2000s, I read a medical research paper discussing the causative factors of Lyme disease. They stated that the severity of the disease was based on two factors, the strength of the pathogen and the strength of the host the pathogen occupies. It's literally a biological tug of war. Through my own clinical findings, I discovered the stronger the occupied host becomes, the weaker the infecting pathogen gets. This is the foundation of the causal chain progression theory. Strengthen the host and allow the body to naturally move towards balance, health, vitality, and optimal performance. This is accomplished by reestablishing three biological influencers: emotional balancing, cellular memory clearing, and correcting nutritional imbalances.

Toxins and pathogens are predominantly influenced by the response of our internal and external environment through the living connective tissue matrix. **The vibration of negative stimuli influences the way our cells replicate and communicate. By simply reprogramming newer positive stimuli using sound, light, frequency, and harmonic vibration, we can directly shift the cellular ecosystem of the host, resulting in a weakening effect of the pathogen.**

Cellular Memory

This one concept I have dedicated my entire professional life to: how to access and clear cellular memory. Before we can clear it, we have to understand what it is and how we can access it. The best way to illustrate cellular memory is to use the example of a concussion. If you have ever had a concussion or seen someone get a concussion, then you know that it is usually associated with a violent trauma of some sort.

During my undergraduate studies in sports medicine and biology, I was exposed to these kinds of injuries regularly. The first concussion is usually the hardest to get. It typically takes a major impact or trauma to cause an initial concussion, and the healing time can be anywhere from a few minutes to several months. Regardless of the healing time, once the injury or trauma occurs, the body stores the memory in its cells. In the future, whenever something similar to the initial trauma happens, the body knows what to do. Subsequent traumas occur more easily because the body holds the memory of the original trauma, is referred to as cellular memory.

What if you experienced other traumas in your life, like your mother being hit by your dad, a classmate making derogatory comments toward you, or a schoolteacher saying that you may not be cut out for college? How will the cellular memory of those memories impact your overall health, vitality, and optimal performance? What if you are exposed to some kind of toxin or infection? How will that impact your cellular communication?

Being able to unlock the cellular memory code is the missing link to most healing modalities and is an emerging area of study in energy and biological medicine. What are the tools necessary to not just access cellular memory but also clear it? **Influencing the biofield influences our nervous system, which influences our chemistry.** Clear the issues in the tissues using positive neurological triggers like sound, light, frequency and vibration. The next two codes will help shed more light on the components of cellular memory.

Vibrational Resonance: The Language of the Body

The body is vibrational in nature. Chemistry is a secondary effect of our vibrational universe processed through the connective tissue matrix. **If we are physical manifestations of our own energetic expression, then it only makes sense to use vibration as a modality for shifting and influencing physiology.**

When you lay in the field of harmonic resonance, only positive chemistry is activated. Based on this concept, I began developing specific vibrational-based therapeutic music in 2007 and have created full body vibrational technology called V.I.B.E.S., or Vibrational Individualized Body Enhancement Systems. They are devices designed to deliver specific harmonic physiological frequencies and vibrations to access a biological phenomenon called full body neurological entrainment, or body hypnosis.

Hypnosis is a process that induces a trance-like state to access different levels of the subconscious to release and reprogram different physiological effects. Hypnosis is mostly considered to influence the brain. As stated previously, we are more than the brain and spinal cord, we are an interconnected network of vibrational materials called microfilaments, microtubules and intermediate tubules that respond to vibrational resonance. Full body neurological entrainment (FBNE) is a highly effective method for quickly, safely and effectively assisting in balancing the body, promoting relaxation, activating healing responses, stimulating the brain, and nervous system balancing, as well as a variety of other physiology optimizing processes.

Water: The Vital Medium for Cellular Activation

Out of all the codes that have been discussed in this chapter, the most significant and profound for obtaining health, wealth, and optimal human performance is understanding the properties of water.

Humans consist of 70% to 90% water, with the other 10% consisting of connective tissue. It is the conductive medium for which the living connective tissue matrix can conduct vibrational resonance through. Inherently, water is not a good conductor as it requires minerals to create a conducive environment. Mineralized water also raises the pH of water. Raising the pH creates a more alkaline medium which, by definition, is more anti-inflammatory. Conversely, stripping minerals from water for the purpose of removing harmful toxins, with all reverse osmosis water systems, creates a liquid that is just as, if not more toxic than the toxins being removed.

Removing minerals from water reduces the conductivity of the water. When conductivity is reduced, it takes on the characteristics of an insulator. Insulating properties reduce the ability to transmit energy, information and vibration between the cells and the surrounding environment.

It comes back to the causal chain progression theory; strengthen the host, and inherently the pathogen will weaken. That same concept works for water. **Raise the vibration of the water and lower vibration; contaminants will not be able to thrive or even exist in that environment.**

There are over 100 trillion cells in the body. Without optimal conductivity to allow neurological impulses to easily move through every tissue, system, and cell of the body, we reduce the ability to receive the effects of vibrational resonance from our environment through the body. Imagine a cooler. The contents inside of the cooler are isolated from the outside environment. This is a good idea for food and beverages. For humans, this is a recipe for inhibiting optimal biological expression.

James Oschman, author of *The Scientific Basis of Energy Medicine*, states that a 10% reduction in hydration results in a reduction in cellular function by one million times.

Disease is a direct effect of a breakdown in optimal cellular communication. Remember the Lyme disease study that stated the severity of the disease is directly proportional to the strength of the host versus the strength of the infection. The stronger the host, the less opportunity there is to allow low vibrational frequencies to enter the energetic field. Statistics show that most senior citizens who "die of natural causes." Have a hydration level of about 40 to 50%. According to Dr. Oschman's statistics, that would result in cellular communication reduction of 4 million times! How many of us could function at our highest expression with our nervous system reduced by that amount? Applying this same statistic to a computer, its coding would become a breeding ground for malware and viruses. Our human computers are no different.

The Key to Optimal Health, Wealth and Vitality is Simply Good VIBES!

The five neurological codes discussed in this chapter are vital doctrines that when understood and applied will open doors of unimaginable human potential. The best place to start is simply drinking highly conductive water. Then review the four other codes and see how you can start making changes in your daily life. If you are looking for technology to help assist with the implementation of these codes in your life, investigate vibrational sound resonance technology as well as therapeutic light, please visit www.bioharmonictechnologies.com for more information.

All of these topics are explained in more detail in my book,

Primal Resonance: Discover the Secrets to Health, Vitality and Optimal Human Performance.

About the Author

Dr. Steven Schwartz

Dr. Schwartz is a visionary technology designer, sound alchemist, and regenerative medicine expert with 20 years of clinical experience, specializing in the advanced treatment of chronic illness, allergies, autoimmune diseases, and emotional imbalances using energy and vibrational healing techniques and technologies.

Dr. Schwartz is the founder of Bioharmonic Technologies, which is a therapeutic music production company that creates music specially designed for shifting and influencing physiology and is the creator of Vibrational Individualized Body Enhancement Systems (VIBES).

He is the author of *Primal Resonance, Discover the Secrets to Health, Vitality and Optimal Human Performance*, which discusses the 10 ways for reversing aging and degeneration using, sound, light frequency, vibration, and the new epidemic in America, chronic systemic inflammation.

Contact Information:
Website: www.bioharmonictechnologies.com
Facebook: @bioharmonictechnologies
Instagram: @bioharmonictechnologies
YouTube: Bioharmonic Technologies
Facebook: @drstevenschwartzdc
Instagram: @drstevenschwartzdc
YouTube: Dr Steven Schwartz DC

75 PERCENT OF THE BRAIN IS WATER

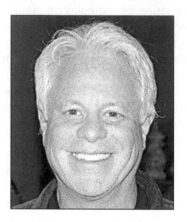

Dr. Terry Rondberg

I have enjoyed a lifetime interest in natural healing and believe that increasing brain function is the cornerstone to helping individuals live a long, happy, and healthy life. In fact, research shows that the body is designed to help all of us achieve this. However, the human body cannot function at 100% of its potential if there is interference in the body. I am an avid lifelong student of correcting nerve interference. I'm also a diplomate of The College of Energy Medicine and The College of Mind-Body Medicine. I developed BioEnergy® an advanced brain-based health care technique that focuses on the sub-occipital muscles that attach directly to the dura mater surrounding the brain stem, which I refer to as the "primary control center" of the human body.

I am excited to share this powerful work with you. This advanced brain-based health care is perfect for people who currently have health problems, because it can provide relief for many painful conditions including back and neck pain, stress, imbalance, instability, and even more where other methods have failed. However, the objective of BioEnergy® is the prevention of sickness, pain, and disease, allowing people to enjoy more vibrant levels of health and wellness without having to get sick or injured in the first place.

The purpose of BioEnergy® is not to diagnose or treat symptoms or disease, which is the domain of Western medicine through its use of drugs and surgery. Instead, our sole purpose is to utilize this advanced healing brain technique to correct interference in the normal flow of energy in the body. We focus on the uppermost part of the cervical spine to optimize the function of the brain—our master control system. This technique can be safely used on virtually everyone.

Almost every culture throughout history has recognized the existence of an all-pervading underlying force that enlivens and integrates the world. In India, this force is known as prana. In Hebrew it is called *ruach*. Followers of Islam call it *Baraka*, and in the Orient, it is known as *qi* or *chi*. This life energy is often described as the "breath of life" because it is considered the vital essence that animates and gives life to the physical form.

When this energy is robust and balanced in an individual, it provides radiance and vitality. When lacking and imbalanced, it leaves one sick, cold, and weak. In the 20th century, Dr. Harold Saxton Burr, a professor at Yale University, was able to measure this rarefied form of matter, conducting many research experiments and publishing many papers on it in the scientific peer-reviewed literature.

Practitioners of BioEnergy® are often MDs, DCs, DOs, acupuncturists, naturopaths, homeopaths, nutritionists, massage therapists, physical therapists, physician assistants, nurses, personal trainers, and estheticians. They use BioEnergy® to complement their work or use it exclusively.

At the core of all-natural healing is the belief that the totality of the Universe is an expression of energy and is connected in a vast, underlying network that nourishes and affects every cell. Some of these connections are visible, like the network of blood vessels within the human body or the waters that connect the rivers of the world. Others are more elusive and can only be felt, like the emotional ties that bind people to one another. Invisible as they may be, they still form potent bonds that can be harder than steel to break.

These underlying vital pathways that link and "feed" everything are seen as absolutely necessary for existence. Just as an arm or leg would weaken and die without a supply of blood and oxygen, so too would our life end if this energy did not circulate within us. In this way, the human being can be seen as a baby nestled in the womb of an energetic universe, being continuously fed through invisible streams of energy. If this connection is severed, the body is no longer able to receive nourishment and its ability to sustain life ceases. The strength of this connection determines our health and well-being on all levels—physical, emotional, and spiritual. When this connection is strong, the body is full of health and vitality. When it is weak, the amount of energy received by the body diminishes, upsetting an individual's physical and psychological health.

The practice of BioEnergy® can produce a profound change in an individual's life. The study of brain health care in the United States is not an education that is readily provided in school or as part of one's normal education. Because of this, coming to terms with that which is invisible often requires opening oneself to a new set of rules and ideas that may be completely foreign to one's established foundation. Even simply accepting the concept of brain health care requires a radical shift in understanding life and oneself, because it also means accepting that we are not isolated entities from the world around us. The realization that our words, actions, and very being affects everyone and everything can stretch the edges of one's conscience so that we feel a greater sense of responsibility for the world around us. However, once this idea is embraced, it can be deeply comforting to feel the limits of endless self-expansion.

In addition to many ancient practitioners of brain health care like energy healing, including Hippocrates, the father of Western medicine, medical researchers within our own time have paved the way for practitioners today to engage in their healing work with confidence. Contemporary scientists such as Dr. Burr, Dr.

Valerie Hunt at UCLA, and Dr. Marilyn Schlitz at the Institute for Noetic Sciences—to name but a few—have conducted peer-reviewed research studies and are published in the scientific literature extensively.

One of the earlier forms of energy healing in the 20th century that inspired me was Dr. Randolph Stone's Polarity Therapy, an open-ended system that utilizes whatever means necessary to establish balance and order in the human energy field. Dr. Stone, who was a chiropractor, naturopath, and osteopath, incorporated bodywork, dietary counseling, exercise, stretches, and changes in thought and lifestyle. With his background as a doctor in three Western forms of medicine, Dr. Stone developed his energy work with a firm foundation in the science of body structure and function. His later explorations in the Eastern arts of energy, including the Ayurvedic medicine of traditional India, traditional Chinese medicine, yoga, and reflexology helped to create a form of bodywork that spanned the range of different approaches from structural to energetic. After extensive research in a variety of medical philosophies and practices, Dr. Stone came to the realization of the existence of certain fundamental principles that tie together all fields of healing. He concluded that all of existence flows from one source and is composed of one universal, energetic substance.

I've been very fortunate to have studied with some of the greatest teachers of contemporary India, including those in the same lineage of Dr. Stone, who spent many years of his life living in India. This has made me even more desirous to bring brain health to you in its clearest, simplest form and *through you*, out to the rest of the world. Having discovered the portal of entry into our energetic system—namely, the suboccipital region of the spine—I feel confident that you will very quickly come to excel in the practice of this unique work.

With the advent of Western science and, in particular, Cartesian thinking, which believes the mind and the body are separate, topics such as vibration and energy flow have not been a big part of everyday conversation about human health for a long time. The emphasis shifted to a "pill for every ill," with dramatic and negative effects becoming the norm. Western science taught us to view the body as solid objects designed to break down. Modern medicine has gone so far as to give diseases Latin names and aggressively treat these diseases by cutting out and medicating various parts of the body. When a person no longer has symptoms, we say that he or she has been cured. Sadly, this is the paradigm of "health" that most people are familiar with today.

BioEnergy® is one of the world's most powerful and advanced brain health care techniques. It has generated outstanding results in the lives of many people and will soon benefit the lives of your practice members. Our clients have reported improved circulation, increased flexibility, increased range of motion, profound stress reduction, deep relaxation, increased energy and vitality, better sleep, self-awareness and insight, a sense of spirituality, better breathing and improved oxygenation, a clearer sense of feeling "balanced," "centered," and "grounded," decreased chronic pain, more optimal skeletal alignment, improved posture, enhanced immune system support through improved detoxification and elimination, release of outdated and negative thought patterns and emotional habits, and enhanced self-esteem.

Athletes report extraordinary results after receiving BioEnergy®. Reported results include more balance during performance, refinement of hand-eye coordination, improvement of mental focus, increased physical and mental endurance, increased flexibility of joints, muscles, and ligaments, faster post-event recovery time, fewer injuries, enhanced power and strength, reduced swelling and edema, and faster tissue healing following injury. Many athletes also insist on receiving BioEnergy® prior to their competition.

What exactly, then, is BioEnergy®? Several important points first need to be made. BioEnergy® is a highly innovative, sophisticated, and integrated fusion of modern Western medicine science and Ancient Eastern healing systems. In my clinic in Southern California, I combine BioEnergy® with whole food nutrition, hydration, and advanced ways of thinking and communicating with the brain that leverage the power of the mind and spirit to promote healing by your body.

Some specific components of BioEnergy® are that:

- It promotes tangible healing results.
- It is a quick and gentle application.
- It is specific to the muscles of the suboccipital area of the upper cervical spine, which directly attaches to the connective tissue covering the brainstem called dura mater.
- It increases the performance of the brain that controls and regulates all functions of your body and mind.

BioEnergy® practice and principles can be combined with nursing, chiropractic, physical therapy, medicine, acupuncture, Ayurveda, massage, and nearly any form of bodywork to enhance its effect. Because this is a clothes-on technique, it can be demonstrated anywhere with anyone. This is a fantastic advantage that helps to create rapport with potential patients. Also, BioEnergy® isn't strenuous to the practitioner like many other forms of bodywork, so it greatly reduces your risk of injury from repetitive motion and muscle strain.

I refer to this as "vibrational" in nature because, first of all, the body is vibrational or energetic in nature, and this brain technique releases chronic tension and interference with the flow of your life energy. Also, BioEnergy® uses a state-of-the-art percussion instrument that applies frequency-specific percussive or vibrational input into the muscles and mechanoreceptors in the upper neck. These receptors tell your brain how you're functioning and direct electrical impulses to your critical brain centers.

Dr. Robert Fulford was an osteopathic physician, considered by many in his own profession, as well as among medical doctors—including Dr. Andrew Weil—as their mentor. He wrote books on energy medicine and was an early pioneer in vibrational healing. After a long and illustrious career, he practiced up to the last week of his life, passing away at the age of 93. Dr. Fulford gave a keynote speech to the American Cranial Academy. He felt a great urgency in delivering his talk and told his closest friends that this message was the last thing he wanted to offer his profession.

The subject of his talk was "The Future of Osteopathy," which concluded with the admonition that "energy healing is the future of medicine." Two days later, having successfully finished his mission, the good doctor passed away.

When someone came to visit Dr. Fulford's office, they would be greeted by a handmade sign on which he had written what he felt to be the key principle of health:

"The human body is comprised of complex streams of moving energy. When these energy streams become blocked or constricted, we lose the physical, emotional, and mental fluidity potentially available to us. If the blockage lasts long enough, the result is pain, discomfort, illness, and distress."

Modern science is beginning to catch up with pioneers such as Dr. Fulford. Thanks to discoveries in the field of quantum physics and neuroscience, we now recognize that the human body is not just a physical structure but is first and foremost composed of bioenergy fields, "complex streams of moving energy." Science can measure electrical currents from the heart with an electrocardiogram, electrical energy from the brain with an electroencephalogram, and a lie detector test picks up energy fields emanating from the skin. Various magnetic imaging devices, night vision instruments, and Kirlian photography can visualize and measure the electromagnetic field surrounding the human body.

For much of the 20th century, our medical culture fostered the idea that only a medical doctor was capable of taking care of a person's health. Fortunately, in the latter part of the 20th century, that notion began to change as more people, including researchers and physicians such as Dr. Fulford, Dr. Randolph Stone, James Oschman, PhD, and Dr. Andrew Weil, came to understand that Western medicine does not have all of the answers with respect to health and wellness. In fact, the most honest medical doctors—among them being Dr. Joseph Mercola, Dr. Mehmet Oz, Dr. Larry Dossey, and the late Dr. Robert Mendelsohn—concede that Western medicine sometimes has no answers and may oftentimes make a person worse.

Scientists are discovering through research that our body seems to be organized in the same way as the Universe, giving credence to the saying, "As above, so below." I will talk more specifically about this in the second module of this course, but for now let me say that I'm certain research will continue to prove we are a microcosm, energetic in nature, of the macrocosm that we call the Universe. Perhaps this is what is meant in the Bible when it is said that we are created in the image of God.

Today, science has come around to accepting the body has a finely tuned energy system that follows nerves and other pathways called meridians. These nerves and meridians interact with a number of more concentrated bioenergy centers called chakras, as well as with a detectable energy field around the body. If energy really does pervade and saturate every cubic centimeter of space throughout the Universe, as the poet Walt Whitman wrote, and eminent physicists such as David Bohm and Albert Einstein informed us, then these "complex streams of energy" are part and parcel of our intimate connection with each other, as well as to everything else that exists.

We believe that this bioenergy flows from "above down, inside out," and that the suboccipital area of the upper neck is a unique portal into the entirety of this complex system. It is also here where stress is often first felt in the body and where interference in the bioenergy system commonly occurs.

There are many factors in our external environment that can have negative effects on our body. Disease-causing pathogens, pollution, toxins, and electromagnetic frequencies not compatible with our nervous systems are a few examples. When an individual's cellular function is negatively altered or compromised over an extended period of time, negative changes often begin. When the cellular level is affected, physical symptoms often appear. The health of the membranes in the cells of your brain is viewed as the first layer of defense before the human body is affected. Knowing the health of your membranes of your brain cells gives us insight into the current and future state of your health. But you might ask, "If we cannot see the cell membranes of our neurons then how can we detect if something is wrong with them?" That is why labs exist. Labs can accurately measure, and we can track and improve your health.

For more information about *BioEnergy Breakthrough* by Dr. Terry A Rondberg, it is available at https://www.goodreads.com/book/show/25623688-BioEnergy®-breakthrough

About the Author

Dr. Terry Rondberg

For over 43 years, Dr. Rondberg has wholeheartedly devoted himself to improving the health and lives of others. For many years he did this as a chiropractic practitioner and educator. Dr. Rondberg was the publisher of *The Chiropractic Journal* for over 25 years, as well as founder and President of the World Chiropractic Alliance. He is the founder and publisher of the *Journal of Vertebral Subluxation Research* and the author of several bestselling books and the patient education book, *Chiropractic First*, which has sold over 3 million copies.

Contact Information:
Email: terry@rondberg.com
Website: www.worldchiropracticalliance.org/
Telephone: 1-800-347-1011

TAKING CHARGE OF THE TIME MACHINE

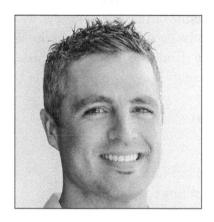

Dr. Tod Pelly

For anyone reading this, it's likely you have a good idea of what stress and time are. They're so common in our normal daily conversation that the two words carry an implied understanding. In a person's everyday life, stress can have different subjective meaning based on how the word is used. For the purpose of this chapter however, we will refer to how it affects an organism and the effects it brings about in that organism. Time has been a very important subject of study in science and philosophy but is decidedly easier to define. It can have a personal intrinsic value due to the human awareness of the limited duration we have upon this earth. In this sense, time is finite and ironically unpredictable.

As a practicing chiropractor, the subjects of stress and time have significant meaning to me and the two are inextricably linked. This has actually become the driving force behind many of my decisions in life and practice over the past few years, and they serve as the basis of most of what I do as a practitioner, husband, friend and father. They're so fundamental to what we do every day that they deserve a deeper look.

In the Westernized world, stress is an epidemic. Roughly 75% of adults between the ages of 20 and 64 report "some levels of stress," and nearly 35% report "extreme stress on a regular basis." This has become such an intense area of discussion within the forums of the World Health Organization that it has declared stress as the epidemic of the 21st century.

What does stress do to us, according the WHO? A shortened list would include (from the head downwards):

o   headaches
o   depression
o   insomnia
o   heartburn
o   weakened immune function
o   rapid breathing
o   high blood sugar
o   increased risk of heart attack
o   high blood pressure
o   stomach aches and digestive issues
o   fertility problems
o   low sex drive
o   erectile dysfunction
o   missed periods
o   tense muscles

If you look at this list, it looks a lot like most of the diseases that are plaguing us daily, driving up the costs of medical expenses and robbing us of our precious human experiences.

In late May of 2018, I experienced my first (and only) panic attack. It was scary. It started with my usual bedtime routine of going through the day's events, my life events, the current state of my family, and where we're headed. It took the typical mental detour into "Life is happening too quickly," and "My kids are growing up too fast," and within a few minutes jumped to "Pretty soon they'll be grown up and I'll be an old man," and "My life is spinning out of control and I'm not enjoying myself at all!"

Time itself seemed to accelerate and all perception of reality began to slip by. My heart was pounding, I was disoriented, I had trouble breathing, and my chest was tight. I sat upright in my bed and did my best to get air into my lungs. I was dripping with sweat and before long, my muscles were so tense they were beginning to cramp. The icy grip of anxiety had taken hold of every conscious thought and it had affected my physical body so much that it felt like I was on a rocket ship, warping through time and headed to oblivion.

Julie, my wife, helped calm me down by getting wet towels to sponge my sweat off and coached me to breathe properly and gain control of my thoughts. Before too long, my feet were back on planet Earth and I was breathing normal oxygen again. The entire experience lasted for only a couple of hours, but it changed me forever. I began asking myself, a guy who is usually well in control of my emotions and physical state, what happened and what did it mean?

As with anything, an experience is only as important as the meaning we assign to it. So, I could just dust myself off and carry on, or I could take this as an opportunity to study myself and find deeper meaning from it. I could push it away or pull it closer—one is easy and the other is an opportunity.

What did it mean to me? What do I do with this experience and how do I feel about it? First of all, it showed me that stress had created a toxic cycle inside my brain that had an impact so powerful that it changed my physiology to the point where I lost my mental tether to reality. It showed me that things only have the meaning I give them, and most importantly, that stress has a profound impact on the perception of time.

After sitting with these thoughts for a while, I had come up with some rules and signposts that would guide my thoughts and decisions from then on. Time seems to move at different rates, and the multiplying factor is stress. When we're "stressed out," or as physiologists call it, "sympathetic dominance," we feel like time moves much more quickly. Stress and time have an interesting relationship in that time seems to stop and stand still when stress is low, and it races faster when we're anxious or under pressure.

Standing on a paddleboard for half an hour in the middle of a calm lake induces quite a different state of physical being than does ironing out final details of an underprepared speech in front of industry peers in 30 minutes. Each carries the same number of seconds, but each gives a much different perception of that time.

Does this mean that stress is bad? Do we live a happier and more complete life without stress? Absolutely not. We need stress. We need it to give us perspective and recalibrate our setpoints so when we do have those precious moments where time seems to stop, we can appreciate them more. Life is built on precious moments and we need to accumulate them in order to feel fulfilled.

How I've come to look at stress and how I discuss it with patients is a little more refined, but the essence is the same.

Stress comes in four forms: physical, chemical, mental and vibrational. When you look at these stresses and the physiologic stress response to them, they become the root of most illness. It should be noted again here that while too much of these four stresses pushes the organism beyond its ideal equilibrium toward disease, too little stress has its own set of issues. We need some stress; it forces growth, but too much stress pushes a system beyond recovery.

When too much stress placed on a bone, it breaks, while not enough stress put on a bone causes fragility and osteoporosis. Too much mental stress causes anxiety and depression, while not enough stress deprives it of growth and development. Eating tainted food can cause disease and sickness, while eating food that has become too sterilized can rob it of the good bacteria, nutrients, and vitamins required to help our bodies grow and gain resistance. Whether it's physical, mental, emotional, chemical, or vibrational stress, we need some of it in order to become stronger people.

Let's look at the brain and how it handles these stresses. How can we help our brains be active and fulfilled while maintaining the right amount of rest and reflection? Is there a way we can get more out of life by understanding and implementing some simple rules around brain health?

As a chiropractor, I feel that turning back time (or at least slowing it down) by dissipating stress on the nervous system is our purpose. Not only is it an important way to look at what we do in the context of helping people live freer lives, if we mentally think of slowing time down by allowing our patient's body and brain to dissipate stress more effectively, and by putting our attention/intention toward that purpose, the outcome can be infinitely more effective. By reducing stress, we slow time down.

Whether it's decreasing physical stress on joints, mental stress on the nervous system, vibrational stress on our various organic systems, or chemical stress of our cells, the role of any practitioner should be the same: to identify and then equilibrate these four types of stresses on our patients so that they can literally slow time down and age better.

As with anything, understanding a problem is the first critical step towards solving it. The first step in the famous 12-step program of Alcoholics Anonymous is admitting there's a problem. Once the problem has been identified, it can be properly addressed. Similar to the 12-step program, admitting that we're powerless is important. We are somewhat powerless over many of the forces that shape our world; trying to force our will on immutable facts might cause more stress and worry than should be reasonably expected. The brain loves to solve problems and find resolutions in neat, simple packages. This is often proven futile and stressful for the brain unless we first realize what we can control and what we cannot.

One of my favorite analogies I share with my patients is the concept of "normal arthritis." Let's say someone has an x-ray done of his knees. The x-ray report will undoubtedly say that there are some degenerative changes/arthritis on the one knee, usually normal for the age of the patient, and some recommendations about course of action might be given for that knee, but none for the good one. This makes perfect sense on the surface. The only problem is that both knees are obviously the same age. So why has one knee "aged" so much faster than the other? I'm sure you've guessed it. The stress on that knee, sustained for a period of time, has accelerated how fast it has aged.

This idea can be applied to different aspects of brain health. A reasonable amount of stress is productive, whereas if the brain is overtaxed for an extended period of time, it begins to fatigue and falter. Memory gets worse, anxiety and depression inevitably increase, creative thoughts and insights become less impactful, and cognition dramatically worsens. Secondary effects on relationships (both personal and interpersonal) are negatively affected, and general enjoyment of life falls off the proverbial cliff.

Continuing with the knee analogy, brain stress can come in the form of trauma or microtrauma. Traumatic brain injuries (concussions) are the equivalent to a blown-out knee from sports activities, whereas excessive wear on a knee would parallel chronic mental stress. Social media, screens, and technology, biologically incompatible electromagnetic frequencies, economic, and social pressures all force their way into our lives and rob us of precious time. They force us to abandon introspective thoughts and make everything else "urgent" and in need of our immediate attention. Identifying these problems, to use the Alcoholics Anonymous analogy, is the first step. Knowing that this is the world we live in and knowing that we can't change many of these facts helps to reduce the frustration around it all and allows us to become more solution focused. Practitioners can then more easily shift toward helping their patients adapt to these stresses more effectively.

My panic attack was the breakthrough I needed to begin shifting my intention with my patients. It was the gift that allowed our practice to evolve to include a wide array of technologies to dramatically reduce brain stress in our patients. While chiropractic care centers around reducing physical and mental stresses, we're now able to incorporate some powerful adjunctive therapies to enhance the innate ability of our patients' bodies to heal themselves mentally, chemically, physically, and vibrationally. With this approach, patient outcomes have dramatically improved and patients report significant improvements in the most basic ways: happiness and life fulfillment.

Whether it's normalizing electromagnetic field frequencies, accelerating tissue responses to healing, or moving a brain from high stress and fatigue to healthy regenerative patterns, the focus of any healthcare practice must shift toward helping its patients process their stresses if they want to slow or reverse aging and improve their overall quality of life.

If a body is more capable of being active, the owner of the body is likely to live a healthier lifestyle and therefore be in better cardiovascular health. A better cardiovascular system has been shown time and time again to improve brain function. It improves mood, coping strategies, and has even been shown to improve standardized test scores in school-age kids. Through proper care and becoming more brain focused, an increasing number of health practitioners are becoming more aware of the role of physical health on mental health. A healthy and happy brain will usually follow a healthy and happy body, and vice versa. Of course, a highly focused and specific chiropractic adjustment delivered to the nervous system is essential to impact brain health but understanding the secondary effects of a better functioning body is important if we ever want to help our patients achieve true happiness and less disease.

About the Author

Dr. Tod Pelly

Dr. Tod Pelly lives with his wife Julie and their two kids, Reid and Kasey, in North Vancouver, Canada. After graduating Magna Cum Laude from Southern California University of Health Sciences in 2005, he practiced and studied the Gonstead Method of Chiropractic in Los Angeles before bringing it back home to Vancouver in 2007. While doing his undergraduate coursework at Simon Fraser University, Dr. Pelly achieved All-American status in Track and Field three times. His diverse background of athletics and academics has put him in a unique position to understand both the mental and physical states of high-level athletes, aspiring athletes, high pressure career-focused executives, and kids with high athletic aptitude.

For more information about Dr. Pelly and his team of dedicated practitioners, please visit www.ThePellyClinic.ca

THE ART OF BALANCE

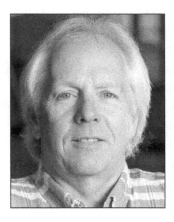

Dr. Tom Lankering

Energy is everything. To optimize the full expression of life energy, it is important to address how the body expresses life energy and the factors that interfere with the full expression of it.

Can you relate to any of these: insomnia, fatigue, anxiety, memory loss, weakened immunity, digestive issues, mood swings, ADD/ADHD, autoimmune conditions, or depression? Why do people develop these conditions? One answer can be explained in three words. They are stress and balance. People experience more stress than they can handle, and it throws them out of balance. When people can handle the stress, they are balanced, and their health is good. When people cannot handle these stresses, they become out of balance and dis-eased.

What are these stresses? What gets out of balance? Let's start with the stresses. Dr. John Brimhall discusses the Triangle of Health. In this situation, think of a triangle. At the center is optimal health. The triangle represents the six major stressors, which interfere with the full expression of our life energy. The points are physical/structural, mental/emotional, and biochemical/nutritional stress. The sides of the triangle represent electromagnetic radiation (EMFs), toxins, and infections/allergies. Our world has become so stressful because we are constantly bombarded by these stresses.

The body strives for balance, a state of physical equilibrium. In the body it is referred to as homeostasis. This is a state that the body strives to achieve. Our bodies are dynamic and constantly in flux.

Allostasis is, "The process by which a state of internal, physiological equilibrium is maintained by an organism in response to actual or perceived environmental and psychological stressors." This is the process that occurs in a living organism. Life is coping with the constant stresses that demand reactions, responses, and recoveries to adapt to the environment. The body constantly deals with the stresses in life. These days, people experience high levels of stress. Many people suffer from low grade chronic stress. It is the accumulation of the six major types of stressors as well as the duration that has accumulated over a lifetime.

Our bodies were designed to go through a stressful event and then be able to recover from it. Today, people don't have time to recover, going from one stressful event to the next. Often, it is hard to tell when one event ends and the next one starts. Chronic stress creates patterns in our bodies, especially in our brains. It interferes with the brain's ability to function and the body's ability to heal. The brain coordinates all of the processes in the body. When the brain is in balance, the body will be in balance. The brain and the nervous system have a dynamic relationship, coordinating how the body copes with internal and external stresses.

What needs to be in balance?

There are three main processes or systems that work to remain in balance. These are striving to stay in balance not only within themselves but also in relation to the other systems. These balancing acts are: the sympathetic/parasympathetic nervous system, the gut/brain connection, and the HPA (hypothalamic pituitary adrenal) axis. One of the main balancing acts is the relationship between the sympathetic and the parasympathetic nervous systems. The sympathetic system is our fight or flight system, our stress system, and our survival system. The parasympathetic system is our recovery system. It is our healing system that governs recuperation, regeneration, digestion, detoxification, and anti-inflammation processes.

Many are stuck in a stress or survival/fight or flight mode. When this imbalance exists, the body cannot heal. It cannot digest, detox, recover, rejuvenate, or recuperate. Chronic stress creates this imbalance, which leads to chronic dis-ease. Another major highway in the body is the gut-brain connection. Stress in the brain affects the gut; conversely, stress in the gut affects the brain. When this connection is out of balance, people can have digestive issues. Some of these symptoms may be obvious, while others may not. For example, foggy thinking, poor memory, or a lack of concentration may all have dysfunctional digestion at the root of the problem.

There is an epidemic of digestive issues such as irritable bowel syndrome, leaky gut, Crohn's disease, and gluten sensitivity, and the list is increasing. One cause of these digestive issues is the body being stuck in the stress mode, compromising the digestive system. When the body is unable to effectively digest, it is an indication that healing is challenged. The brain is stuck in a brain wave pattern that is not conducive to digestion and healing.

Another aspect of the body being out of balance deals with the HPA axis. The components of this axis are the hypothalamus, pituitary, and adrenal glands. The adrenal glands are the cornerstone of the endocrine system. A metaphor is the adrenal glands are the "push" and the thyroid gland is the "pull" that drives the pump in the body. The other players on the team are the glands of the endocrine system. When the adrenals get tired, the rest of the team has to pick up the slack.

This is analogous to when one player on a basketball team cannot play up to their potential, and other players on the team need to pick up the slack. It is only a matter of time until the domino effect occurs, and the rest of the team loses the ability to perform its duties. Adrenal fatigue or exhaustion are epidemic in our society. Chronic stress has taken its toll. This takes its toll on the HPA axis because this pathway affects the balance of neurotransmitters. Basically, when there is stress in the body, it affects the mind. When there is stress in the mind, it affects the body.

When people get sick, they want to find out what they "have." Often, doctors will give them a name for what they are experiencing without addressing the cause of the symptoms or conditions. The bottom line is that if people want to put a name on what they are suffering from, it could be called an "accumulated stress disorder." It is important to realize that sickness and illness do not just happen. They usually result from an accumulation of violations of Universal laws and the body tries to tell us that something is wrong. Many people will not heed their body's messages until a crisis point is reached. For some, it may be too late as their bodies may have gone beyond their capacities to heal.

Yet with the miraculous body that we have, it is never too late to expect miracles. There is no limit on the body's healing capacity providing that we remove the interferences and provide the right foods and resources that the body needs. The body is very resilient yet extremely sensitive.

The subconscious or "other than conscious" part of the brain plays a powerful role in our healing and functioning in this world. Our perception of our bodies plays a tremendous role in our place in the world. We are more than just a bag of bones. Think of it this way to start. If a car mechanic were to take a car apart and lay all of the pieces out, he could take those pieces, put them back together, start up the car, and drive off. But if now we were to take a person apart and spread those parts about, would you be able to put that person back together again and expect them to walk out of the room? Of course not! So, we realize that there is an energy that exists within our bodies.

Quantum physics and quantum biology demonstrate that we are really more than physical structures. We are actually energetic beings! Even though these different systems have been addressed, it is important to realize that these systems work together as an energy force; they are all one. The body does not work in isolation. There are vast networks and interrelationships throughout the body and within each of these highways in the body. What affects one part of the body will have a ripple effect throughout the body (and the world).

This is a simplified overview. The constant and numerous interactions and functions in the body are mindboggling. It is fortunate that we don't have think about any of this as the body does this all on its own. Our most important responsibility is to clear the body of interferences and toxins. When we do this, the vitalistic wisdom of the body performs miracles every second.

So, how do we do this? While everything is energy, we can control or manage our life energy with conscious thought. Our conscious thought has an immense impact on our subconscious thought. We need to realize that we do have choice, and that choice plays a big role in recovering from stress. Even though the subconscious and the autonomic nervous system coordinate bodily functions, we have the power to choose what we focus on. Once we have awareness, we can then make choices. Our conscious thoughts can focus on and make changes to what we think about. What we think about, we can bring about.

The biggest choice we have is to do something. Even choosing not to do something is a choice. We can choose what we focus on. Having tools to reinforce our decision-making process can be very powerful. Our thoughts lead to our beliefs, which lead to our actions.

What are the best choices to make? They are the choices that will lead to the best chance for health and survival as well as leading to the better good for all. If we function at a lower vibrational frequency, then we make decisions which will not have as much of a positive effect. The first place to start that will have the greatest impact is with the brain.

Brain fitness is key to better health. When we get the brain in balance, the rest of the body comes into balance. The main pathways in the nervous system which lead to the brain are the muscle spindles along the spine, the joint receptors in the spine, the cerebellum, the brain stem, eyes, and ears. A healthy brain shows up with the muscles balanced. Healthy posture is one of extension and relaxation. An imbalanced brain correlates with a posture of flexion and tension.

Chiropractic adjustments actually create pattern interruptions that impact brain waves. These stimulations create pattern interruptions in the nervous system, which can influence the brain to change its brain wave patterns. Neuroplastic changes and new responses occur in the brain. Structural distortions are actually caused by dysfunctional brain wave patterns. Balancing the brain brings the body to ease. Chiropractic adjustments are a very powerful tool to impact the brain. Many people think of chiropractic as "popping and cracking" the bones back into place because they have a pinched nerve that causes pain. Current research indicates that pain comes from the brain. Pain functions as messages to indicate a dysfunction or disease exists. Restoring a balance of brain waves creates ease in the body.

Light and sound are very effective energies to stimulate changes in the brain. BrainTap, developed by Dr. Patrick Porter, is a technology that uses a headset with eye lights and earphones. By using light, binaural beats, isochronic tones, guided imagery, and music, brain waves can be entrained to new patterns. This creates a healthy balance of the brain waves which are mainly beta, gamma, alpha, theta, and delta. There are over 800 programs, which create neuroplastic changes in the brain. The mechanism works just like looking in the flames of a fire. We become mesmerized because our brain adapts to the light frequencies. Sound has a similar impact on the brain. Photo biomodulation or low-level cold laser therapy is valuable in stimulating neuroplastic changes.

Emotional release is also critical to optimizing the full expression of life energy. Emotions have energy—lots of energy. If I were to ask you to show me what happiness, anger, fear, or any other emotion looks like; you would show me an energetic pattern in your body. When we experience emotional events that have so much energy associated with them, they can create distortions in our bodies. These distortions remain until the neuro-emotional complexes are reset. Our emotions are stored in the limbic system of the brain. They are the subconscious emotions; we are not consciously aware of them. Emotions control our thoughts and actions 95% of the time. Neuro-Emotional Technique (NET), developed by Dr. Scott Walker, resets the body and brain to neutralize the impacts that emotions manifest in the body.

The Koren Specific Technique, developed by Dr. Tedd Koren, enables one to determine where energy blockages are occurring in the body. One is then able to make adjustments to facilitate optimal expression of the life force in the body. Detoxification is crucial to balancing the body. If you pour dirt in your gas tank, the car is not going to run well (if at all). Heavy metals, environmental toxins, and congested acupuncture meridians all need to be addressed. Methods to detox include ion foot baths, nutritional cleanses, far-infrared saunas, and homeopathic remedies.

Hemp oil is effective at balancing the body. A broad spectrum of cannabidiols and full entourage of terpenes support the endocannabinoid system. The ECS system supports the parasympathetic system. This sacred plant has the ability to restore and purify our bodies. Hemp oils that contain CBG may be very effective to support and maintain the brain to achieve balance.

Good nutrition is critical to optimizing our health. Vitamin supplements are often necessary because either our bodies have been so out of balance or because the nutritional demands placed on our bodies from all of the stresses cannot be met. It is essential to consume organic food and supplements. Whole food concentrated supplements, which have a pre-digested enzyme delivery system ensure that your body absorbs the proper nutrients it needs.

The first step to implement these practices is to become aware and conscious of what we think, what we put into our bodies, and what we do. Making better choices will eventually lead to a healthier life that will be easier to maintain, as opposed to a life of disease that is painful and takes much effort to change. The choice is yours. Make a decision to be healthier. You can become a better version of yourself. When you can be the best that you can be, then you can enjoy life's journey and you can help others to improve the quality of their lives.

About the Author

Dr. Tom Lankering

Dr. Lankering earned his Doctor of Chiropractic degree from Palmer College of Chiropractic and his Bachelor of Science from the State University of New York (SUNY) at Albany. He worked his way through chiropractic school as a ski instructor and piano player in Aspen, Colorado.

In 1984, Dr. Tom established Lankering Chiropractic and Wellness Clinic in Aspen, Colorado. He has maintained his practice in the Roaring Fork Valley since then. The emphasis of his bio-energetic practice has been a holistic approach utilizing high-tech with high-touch in addressing the stresses that people face and helping them manage their stress to restore their health. The focus of his work is brain-based wellness. This work improves brain fitness by implementing BrainTap technology, nutrition, detoxification, photo biomodulation, emotional release techniques, and other advanced chiropractic methods. Dr. Lankering is a certified Brimhall Technique practitioner and a graduate of the Koren Specific Technique training. He also works extensively with the Neuro-Emotional Technique.

In 2005 Dr. Lankering was the Colorado Presidential Chiropractor of the Year. He also served as the president of the Colorado Chiropractic Association. He has been the host and producer of his television show "Healthy Lifestyles" on the Grassroots TV station in Aspen, Colorado since 1995.

During the winters you can find him on the slopes of Aspen Mountain as a ski ambassador and during summer as a volunteer forest ranger with the Forest Conservancy in the White River National Forest.

Contact Information:
Website: www.lankeringchiropractic.com
Facebook: www.facebook.com/lankeringchiropractic.com

THE BRAIN TRIFECTA

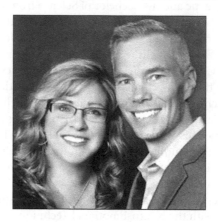

Drs. Bridget and Karl Krantz

It was a beautiful day to be at the ski hill. Some of our kids were ski racing, while others were just out skiing for fun. Having seven kids, they were all over the ski resort, but most of them were quite accomplished skiers. Karl and I were having a great time visiting with other parents and enjoying the large fire pit and view of the ski hills. Out of the blue and off to the side, I heard several adults make a loud "ooh" sound, the one you make when you watch something that had to have hurt. I turned around and saw a limp, almost lifeless body sliding down the hill facedown.

My motherly instinct kicked in and I knew it was one of my own children. I started running towards the ski hill yelling at Karl, "Avery is hurt!" He thought I was overreacting, and no way could it have been one of ours. When I finally got to the bottom of the hill, I found Avery walking away stunned, not knowing where he was going. I yelled his name and he turned around for me to see the blood on his face and the total confusion in his eyes. I knew we needed to go straight to the ski patrol.

After asking Avery several questions, we knew something

wasn't right. He could answer basic questions like how many siblings he had, but when we asked him what we had just asked, he went blank. They ended up putting a neck brace on and backboarded him as we waited for the ambulance ride to the hospital. Our lives were going to change, yet we still didn't know the full impact of it at that point.

Avery was a trick skier, and that afternoon he had been doing backflips off a jump. He had landed dozens of them and those flips were second nature. But this ski hill was different; the jump wasn't high enough. Avery didn't get enough height and halfway through his rotation, his ski tips caught the edge of the jump, stopping his momentum and whipping him 10 feet down on his head. Of course, everyone asks if he had been wearing a helmet, but in our lives, helmets are a must. I tell people my kids can ski naked, but not without a helmet!

After a day in the hospital and countless tests and x-rays, he went home with instructions to rest for a few days before resuming normal activities. But over the next few weeks, he demonstrated short-term memory loss, personality changes (or lack of personality), and struggles in therapy. He couldn't go on drives without wearing an eye mask because it was too bright. One therapist even said his eye focusing skills were like that of a 60-year-old. I would get calls from salesclerks saying my son was "lost" and he couldn't remember where I was or that I told him I was going next door into the grocery store. After a few weeks of trying to get back into the swing of things at school, they called to say he was a "different person" and struggling, and maybe that he should finish the 8th grade at home to recover. Normal life activities were no longer an option.

High school came with academic accommodations and its own struggles. He couldn't remember where he put things or certain assignments. We would look at home for his backpack for over 30 minutes because he couldn't remember where he put it when he walked in the door. He looked normal on the outside, but the struggle was real inside. Some teachers couldn't understand and didn't like giving him open notes and extra time. They didn't believe he really had any issues. On the outside, he didn't look like he needed any special accommodations. His own frustrations were a struggle too. He felt defective. Sometimes tears would well up in his eyes because he was so frustrated that his brain didn't work like it did before. He would realize when he forgot something or didn't have the same level of coordination for sports.

Karl is a chiropractor and I am a naturopath. We have worked with many clients in regard to brain health, including concussions, brain trauma, anxiety, depression, ADHD, cerebral palsy, autism, and more. But this was up-close and personal; this was our own child. We did everything we knew, plus more. We learned and researched everything out there and tried it all. We wanted to approach this from every angle possible. And being in the natural health care field, that was the route we trusted we would go.

How can chiropractic help with brain health? How could I help my son? Karl, had over 20 years of experience as a chiropractor and I knew I could help him as I've helped hundreds over the years. In addition to the severe concussion, Avery was also diagnosed with severe whiplash. His x-ray from the ER showed a significant subluxation of his top two vertebrae.

It immediately brought to mind a patient from 18 years prior named Alex (of which I have permission to tell his story). Alex came to me at age nine. He had an extremely traumatic birth. He was born lifeless; no heartbeat and not breathing. Amazingly, he was revived yet suffered significant brain injury. He was diagnosed with cerebral palsy, autism, and a full spectrum of other cognitive disorders. When we first met, he was known to be profoundly violent, would not make eye contact with anyone, and was completely nonverbal.

Carefully but quickly, I examined his neck based on his birth history and lack of patience, because I knew I could not do a full workup on him. I palpated his neck and felt the top vertebrae (the atlas) to be grossly misaligned. To this day, it is the worst subluxation (misalignment) I've ever felt! I only had one chance to adjust him since Alex was fighting to get off the table as his aides and mom held him in place and tried to comfort him. I proceeded to adjust his atlas.

It was incredible! Not only the movement of the vertebrae, but most profoundly what took place next. He immediately went limp... relaxed on the table, took a big deep breath, made direct eye contact with me, and said his very first word: "Good!" All of us were immediately moved to tears for the miracle that had taken place. To this day, 25 years later, I still have the privilege of caring for Alex on a regular basis. His life has forever changed with chiropractic care.

But why did this happen? Multiple studies demonstrate the benefits of chiropractic care on the brain and how it can enhance the communication and expression of life throughout the body. One study in particular from Sherman College of Chiropractic shows that adjustments of the cervical spine can positively affect the brain. Repeated EEG studies show an improvement on the central nervous system, specifically four primary brain waves: beta, alpha, theta, and delta. Most significant was the improvement of the alpha waves, which are responsible for a great degree of relaxation and healing for the body.

So with the experience and knowledge I've gained over all these years, I knew Avery's brain recovery was quite dependent on chiropractic care and realized it would be an integral part of his healing. Like Alex, I needed to release the extreme pressure and tension that was on his cervical spine to ensure proper brain expression and healing through the nervous system. After his care began, we noticed slow but steady changes in his spine as well as his cognitive function.

The most extensive part of his injury was to the frontal lobe, or the prefrontal cortex. This is where personality, expression, behavior, decision-making, memory, attention, emotional responses, and other functions occur. It further made sense why chiropractic helped Avery and Alex when a 2016 study from Denmark was published showing an average improvement of prefrontal cortex function by 20% following chiropractic spinal manipulations. (Neural Plasticity Journal, 2016).

In addition to chiropractic care, I always feel that part of my responsibility of caring for a patient is to build the right team. What team? The team of providers that is needed to facilitate optimum improvement in the patient's health (even when it's our own son). Part of Avery's team included craniosacral and massage therapy which aided in his recovery by further releasing pressure off the spinal cord and associated muscles.

We also knew that nutrition and gut health are a huge factor for the brain. Since we were not comfortable with conventional medications and felt they had not yet shown much benefit, we looked to nutrition to reduce inflammation and protect the brain. Along with curcumin, Vitamin D and creatine, and essential fatty acids in the form of fish oils are some of the natural compounds with potential therapeutic benefits in the treatment of brain injuries. DHA, EPA, flaxseed oil, and lecithins are all helpful oils to lower inflammation and assist with the function of cell membranes. The human brain is about 60% fat, so essential fatty acids are crucial for the brain's integrity and ability to perform. If someone has a poor diet and lower physical activity, often supplementation with enzymes, probiotics, and nutrition are necessary to start and maintain the healing response. For example, all eight B vitamins are crucial for brain health and function. Not only is nutrition important for brain injuries, but we also find its importance in mental health.

There is a strong physical and chemical connection between the mind and digestive system that involves two-way communication. Some people now call the gut and its millions of neurons in its lining the "second brain." Not only does it move food through our system and nourish our body, but the gut sends and receives impulses, records experiences, and responds to emotions. Just like stress can cause digestive disorders, irritations in the digestive tract may trigger mood changes. Research is finding a growing number of people who have bowel problems may also develop anxiety or depression over time.

According to the American Psychological Association, the bacteria in our gut produces neurochemicals that our brain uses for tasks like learning, memory, and overall mood regulation. Serotonin is known as a contributor to feelings of well-being and happiness. It is now known that 90% of the body's serotonin is produced in the gut, yet it is dependent on healthy gut bacteria. So if you are struggling with brain injuries or even anxiety and/or depression, be sure to address your gut health and choose wisely what you put into your body. Besides prebiotics and probiotics, there are many excellent nutritional options to help heal the gut and speed recovery. It is very rewarding to see clients get off medications, with their doctor's approval, after working with us on their natural healthcare journey.

But just as important as good organic food and nutrition is to the body and brain, avoiding certain bad choices are just as relevant. Health consequences can be significant when the gut bacteria is out of balance or damaged. The Standard American Diet is full of highly processed foods that are low in fiber and full of chemicals, sugars, and bad fats. Other things that can damage the gut are antibiotics, other medications, alcohol, pesticides on food, and stress.

With any type of healing, a person also needs to deal with their emotions. Research shows that over two-thirds of us are living in constant stress that we can actually feel in our bodies. Our bodies were not designed to deal with long term levels of high, chronic stress. Research suggests that stress also can bring on or worsen certain symptoms or diseases. According to WebMD, 43% of all adults suffer adverse health effects from stress and 75% to 90% of all doctor visits are for stress-related ailments and complaints. Stress truly needs to be dealt with and overcome to obtain and maintain better health. There are many emotional outlets and ways to help with stress. Meditation, exercise, and a good diet are all crucial.

There is a huge mind/body connection and the ACE (Adverse Childhood Experience) Study shows that childhood trauma has a direct association with health and social problems across the lifespan. (www.cdc.gov/ace/) According to the study, children who experienced specific adverse emotional experiences were prone to many health and social problems that continued into adulthood. Ninety five percent of our brain works on the subconscious level, which automatically reacts to situations and stored behavior. By working with emotions and breaking down subconscious barriers, emotional and physical balance can be restored.

There are many healing modalities that can change your life. A few are BrainTap, Quantum Neuro Reset Therapy (QNRT), faith/prayer, energy work, Emotion Code, aromatherapy, The Healing Code, Emotional Freedom Technique, and so much more. Find something that resonates with you and find someone who knows what they are doing and who is well trained. Working with emotions can be very beneficial, yet delicate. Sometimes you cannot physically heal or truly be pain free until you deal with any stuck subconscious emotions.

It was about six months after the accident when Avery called us to check in. He made a joke and we all laughed. After we hung up, I cried tears of joy. It was the first time since the injury that he showed any personality—his personality. He was going to be okay. Today, Avery is a successful college student with exceptional grades and lots of friends.

The brain is amazing. It's resilient. Give it what it needs, and it will heal. But if you choose to deprive it with poor diet, no exercise, lack of self-care and self-love, you will decline. Your brain has neuroplasticity; it has the ability to change continuously throughout an individual's life. It takes time and work, but it pays endless returns. And you can do it! The Brain Trifecta is healing yourself with chiropractic care, nutrition, and emotional work. You have the power to create your own success. Your body and brain want to heal, they want to thrive, and they want to be happy.

About the Author

Drs. Bridget & Karl Krantz

Bridget Krantz is a nationally board-certified naturopathic doctor with the American Naturopathic Medical Certification Board. She owns Improved Wellness, LLC in Madison, WI. She is also a board-certified natural health care practitioner and member of the American Association of Drugless Practitioners. She cares for people of all ages and offers a personalized health plan using nutrition, homeopathics, herbs, and essential oils. With her advanced training, she has been certified in QNRT (Quantum Neuro Reset Therapy) and MFT (Morphogenic Field Technique).

Bridget works alongside her husband, Karl, who is a Chiropractor. Her seven kids are growing up fast and she just celebrated the birth of her first grandbaby.

Dr. Karl Krantz is a chiropractor in Madison, Wisconsin. He has been in practice since 1994, helping clients from newborns to those over 100 years old. He also has an advanced certification in nutrition through the State of Wisconsin. His wife, Bridget Krantz (a board-certified naturopathic doctor), practices alongside him.

Dr. Krantz is the personal chiropractor for multiple CEOs of national and international corporations. He has also been a presenter/speaker of health and wellness to multiple corporations both small and large, such as Land's End and Electronic Theater Controls. He welcomes the opportunity to speak at your corporation/event or help guide you on your own personal journey of health.

Contact information:
Email: BridgetKrantzND@gmail.com
Facebook: https://fb.me/BridgetKrantzND
Websites: www.improved-wellness.com
                   www.madisonbrain.com/
Email: drlkarlkrantz@gmail.com
Website: www.genesis-chiro.com
Genesis Chiropractic Center, SC
8333 Greenway Blvd., Ste. 140
Middleton, WI 53562
Telephone: (608) 836-8080

GIVE OUT OF YOUR OWN ABUNDANCE

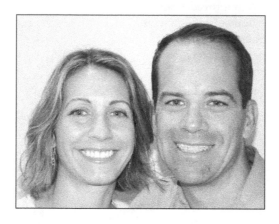

Drs. Deron & Jennifer Jester

"The sole meaning of life is to serve humanity."
-Leo Tolstoy

Sometimes we choose the path we will take in life, and sometimes the path chooses us. Almost twenty years ago we were both chosen to become chiropractors and lead a life of service. We were both drawn to the chiropractic profession because it is rooted in the principles of living with a lasting purpose, loving service to others, and giving out of our own abundance. The treatment performed by most chiropractors includes human contact using our hands to deliver a chiropractic adjustment. There is an exchange of energy between the doctor and the patient, which results in healing. Every specific adjustment is intended to release the healing potential within. When the vertebra are adjusted and the nervous system is awakened, there is an increase flow of energy from the body to the brain and from the brain back to the body, thus reconnecting the natural functioning within. When the body functions properly as it was designed to since conception and birth, the body will heal and life is restored at the cellular, tissue, and system levels within. Since birth, the human frame is forever bombarded with physical, chemical and emotional stressors. As doctors and skilled technicians in the art of the adjustment, it is our duty to neutralize the stress within our patients' bodies, so they have a chance to be healthy and thrive.

The miracles that our profession is known for became a calling for us to truly help patients not only feel better but heal better. The culture surrounding our profession to this day hasn't changed, and in the years since we both graduated from chiropractic school, we have never waivered in our focus on helping others live their best life. The truth as we have come to know it is that living a life of service is a life well spent. Helping others is the secret to living a life that not only brings us greater happiness, health, and prosperity, but above all, meaning.

"We make a living by what we get;
we make a life by what we give."
-Winston Churchill

Deron:

In 1998 while living in Boston, I was invited to a philosophy seminar in Atlanta Georgia called Dynamic Essentials. At that point in my life, I had never been to a chiropractor and knew little about what a chiropractor did. I listened for three days to doctors who spoke about their amazing lives filled with passion, prosperity, and purpose. It was clear that the top practitioners were leading these enchanted lives of loving service to their communities, all the while raising healthy families under this thing called "the chiropractic lifestyle." It became clear that chiropractic was much more than a 9-5, job but instead it was a model for living a fulfilled life. I tried to share my excitement with Jennifer back home. I wanted her to experience the same shift that I had that weekend. Understandably, she couldn't grasp how I had become so excited in such a short period of time and wasn't sure about this "chiropractic lifestyle" I spoke so passionately about.

It was at that seminar where I received my first chiropractic adjustment, which I thought was amazing. I remember smiling and giggling through the whole two-minute experience, trying to hold back my excitement. It was that weekend that I was introduced to a principled doctor practicing in Boston and I returned to begin my journey by becoming an invested chiropractic patient. Eventually, I worked for this doctor as a chiropractic assistant in his office and applied to a chiropractic school in Georgia where my journey had begun earlier that same year.

Jennifer:

When Deron returned from his trip to Atlanta so excited and energized about the idea of applying to chiropractic school, I tried to share his excitement, but the truth was I didn't really get it. Like him, I had never been to a chiropractor and was never introduced to that particular philosophy of health.

While in Boston, I was working for a large mutual fund investment firm, and thought I was content to continue this career path in finance until I suffered an injury while training for the Boston Marathon in 1999 that changed everything. Deron had begun working for a local chiropractor to gain experience before his chiropractic college program began, and after my training injury worsened, he pleaded with me to come into the office and see the doctor. I sat in this chiropractor's office and told him all about my symptoms, and he listened patiently. Then he asked me two very simple questions that changed the way I thought about the function of the human body forever. First: "What do you think caused your body to experience this pain?" Second: "Do you want to correct the problem or simply cover up the symptoms?" It was the first time I really began to think about how my body functioned and not just about how my body felt. With the help of this chiropractor's care, I was able to run the entire 26.2-mile Boston Marathon without any pain.

As an athlete growing up, I was always interested in the body and performance, and I devoured information and articles on nutrition and exercise. However, when Deron and I moved together to Atlanta for him to attend chiropractic college, while I now supported him completely, I still had every intention of continuing my career in finance. That was until one day while sitting in our apartment when I was listening in (as I often did), to his study group and chimed in with a proclamation that, "I love what you guys are learning. If I could do it all over again, I think I would become a chiropractor." To which Deron immediately replied, "Jen, you are only 25 years old; you have time. If you want to pursue a career in chiropractic, then you should do it." I applied to the program shortly after that day and was accepted. This began our journey together to dedicate our lives to the service of others, to help people who are suffering regain their health and function and live their best life.

After getting married and graduating from chiropractic school, our first goal was to find a thriving community to serve. We found just that in West Chester, Pennsylvania (Deron's hometown). Once we established our practice, it became our next goal to help serve as many people as possible and help our neighbors discover the health and wellness benefits of a chiropractic lifestyle. Our purpose and mission statement is *"To serve the members of our community with lifetime chiropractic care and wellness education for a healthier, happier, more productive life."*

Chinese Proverb:

If you want happiness for an hour, take a nap.
If you want happiness for a day, go fishing.
If you want happiness for a month, get married.
If you want happiness for a year, inherit a fortune.
If you want happiness for a lifetime, help somebody else.

Human beings are actually hardwired for service. We don't have to look far to find the research that proves we receive joy from helping others. Giving out of our own abundance has been scientifically proven to stimulate pleasure centers in our brain, releasing the same chemicals and hormones that are released when we are feeling all kinds of joy and love, like serotonin, epinephrine, oxytocin, dopamine, and endorphins.

Sometimes we don't even need to be the person who actually provides service to feel the joy. There was a story that went around a few years back about a New York City police officer that, on a cold November night, noticed a homeless man without any socks or shoes to keep his feet warm. As bystanders gathered to watch, the officer asked the man his shoe size and ducked into a nearby store to buy the man a pair of warm socks and shoes. The display of caring was caught on camera and viewed close to a million times, proving that people love, not only to help others, but also love to witness others giving and serving out of their own abundance.

We are also hardwired for connection. However, this feels harder than ever in today's society as technology, the hectic pace of life, and changing societal norms disconnect us from each other. Engaging in more giving and service can help all of us regain that bond that we seek with others in our community. We are all literally starving for connection. When we give of ourselves to another, we connect with that person, whether it's giving our time, our energy, our expertise, our skills, or our kindness we can't help but become interconnected on some level. This is equally healing and joyful for the giver as it is for the receiver; according to Newton's Third Law: For every action, there is an equal and opposite reaction. By giving joy, we receive joy.

There are five simple rules to help make giving out of your own abundance part of your life so you can experience all of the connection, love, happiness, health, prosperity, and fulfillment that a life of service can provide.

Rule #1 Find Your Purpose and Your Passion

Your purpose is your why? Why are you inspired to help people? For us, our purpose simple, TO SERVE. Then, your mission is the how. How can you use your passion to make that purpose come to life?

Deron:

A couple of years ago, I received an invitation to accompany a group of doctors to the Dominican Republic to help bring the message of health and healing through chiropractic care to some of the most underserved communities on the island. It was such a joy to bring my purpose of helping people live better lives and my passion for adjusting the spine to allow optimal brain and nervous system function to all of the deserving people we met. Locally, we've offered similar services to the Salvation Army as well as in-office services to those unable to pay in order to ensure we reach members of our community with loving service with the intention and outcome of circle-circle, so that they can in return give to others.

Rule #2 Give for Their Highest Good, Not Yours

We had an experience several years back in our office when we decided to do a food drive during the holidays to help a local food bank. We wrapped a big box and made a sign to letting our patients know that we were collecting all types of non-perishable food.

Jennifer:

After the first week the box was really filling up, and I felt so good as I called the food bank to let them know that we'd be bringing in a donation. They thanked me, but also politely asked if it was possible for us to collect toiletries and household items instead of food. They were almost overstocked with food, but in great need of these other items. Initially I felt a bit disappointed... but I soon realized the donations weren't about what we collected, but rather collecting something in need.

Rule #3 Give to Those Who Are Ready to Receive... Be Patient with the Rest

Most of the time, patients who seek our care are ready to make a health shift in their life. They are ready for a natural health solution that can help them feel better, heal better, and be healthier. But every now and then we meet a patient who just isn't ready to make a change. The greatest challenge is when a person who desperately needs our services and help but does not accept our recommendations and they do not follow through with care. They will never know the amazing benefit of their healing potential from within. What is it with their internal wiring and mindset that interferes with their openness for help? We approach every new patient with our best intention, tell them what they need to hear, and serve them the best we can.

Jennifer:

We are fortunate to see so many patients get fantastic results, allowing them to more fully engage in their enjoyment of life, that it is easy for us to believe that everyone is ready to make that kind of change. The reality is that some people aren't ready to change. Maybe they are concerned about how much time it will take or they're hesitant about making the kind of lifestyle modifications necessary. Whatever the case may be, it has been very freeing for me to realize that instead of getting stuck in frustration, I can let them go with love, focus on those that are ready and willing, and let those who are not yet ready know that I will be there for them if and when they become ready for change.

Rule #4 Set Boundaries

When you find a passion for giving and service, it can be very easy to over-extend yourself because of your enthusiasm to help people. Helping people feels good, but when you overextend yourself, the good feelings can disappear.

Deron:

Early on in practice, I was so excited by the chance to help each and every patient that I would stay late, work on weekends, and even take time on holidays to meet a patient in the office. I missed family meals, bedtime for my kids, quality time with Jennifer, swim meets, soccer games, and even sacred holidays. I quickly realized that in order to fully engage in serving my patients to my highest standards, I had to have time to completely disengage from seeing patients in the office. Having time to connect with my family and recharge my own battery helps me serve more and serve better.

Rule #5 Be Willing to Gratefully Receive in Return

When we align our purpose and passion with our profession, prosperity inevitably follows. Over the past 15 years, we have built a thriving practice that is able to serve thousands of people a year, and none of that would be possible if the practice wasn't profitable. Early on in our practice, we almost felt bad collecting a fee from patients. We knew we had to, or our practice would shutter, but it was hard for us to align the act of giving and serving with receiving as well.

We found that patients wanted to give us something in return, and whenever we tried to give away our services, some energetic imbalance seemed to occur. The patient would disappear only to return and tell us they didn't feel right that we had given them a discount or something for free. We find that our relationship with those we serve is the soundest when we are able to gratefully receive in return.

Final Thoughts...

Mahatma Gandhi once said, "The best way to find yourself is to lose yourself in the service of others." Making serving out of our own abundance an anchor in our lives has helped us create a life that is filled with happiness, health, and prosperity. It has given us a sense of purpose, meaning, and connection to our patients and community. Serving others can be contagious... in a great way. You never know when one small act of kindness or gift of service can trigger a cascade of others and result in a show of humanity at its finest. A wise man once said, "A rising tide lifts all boats."

About the Author

Drs. Deron & Jennifer Jester

Dr. Deron Jester:

Dr. Deron Jester is the founder and director of Jester Family Chiropractic, a wellness practice in West Chester, Pennsylvania. He has an undergraduate degree in Biology from St. Lawrence University and his Doctor of Chiropractic from Life University in Atlanta. In 2016, he was awarded the prestigious *Chiropractor of the Year* award by The Master's Circle, and international professional organization. Recently, Dr. Deron received the title of Certified Chiropractic Wellness Practitioner. This certification enables him to incorporate specific nutrition, exercise, chiropractic and rehabilitative programs to serve patient's evolving health and wellness needs.

He specializes in working with patients with all types of cases including degenerative spinal issues, athletes and sports injuries, personal and auto injuries, work-related injuries, pre- and post-natal spinal needs, pediatric spinal conditions, and geriatric-specific spinal issues. He is passionate and committed to empowering people to reach their optimal level of health and function and maintain peak performance throughout their lifetime.

Dr. Deron lectures regularly in the community and to corporate groups on topics as diverse as stress reduction, improved job productivity, disease and injury prevention, and optimal health and wellness strategies. When not in the office serving patients, he enjoys participating and leading rides for his local cycling club, cooking, traveling, skiing, hiking, camping, and family time spent with his wife, Jennifer, and their two children, Caroline and Nathan, and Labrador retriever, Dakota.

Dr. Jennifer Jester:

Dr. Jennifer Jester is the co-founder of Jester Family Chiropractic. She graduated from Bucknell University with a Bachelor of Arts Degree in Economics. She went on to obtain her Doctorate in Chiropractic from Life University. Dr. Jennifer is currently pursuing advanced education and certification in functional medicine to help serve patients suffering with chronic conditions and those looking for a whole-body approach to health and wellness.

In their practice, Dr. Jennifer is passionate about helping women and children and regularly treats women for pre- and post-natal spinal concerns, children from infants to teenagers, and women of all ages.

She enjoys volunteering for local charities, non-profit organizations, and volunteering in her community. She is active and makes her own health a priority through running, fitness training and functional exercise. She also enjoys reading, cooking, travelling, skiing, hiking, camping, and family time with Deron, their two children, and Labrador Retriever.

Contact Information:
Website: www.jesterchiropractic.com
Facebook: www.facebook.com/JesterChiropractic
Instagram: www.instagram.com/jesterchiro

THE QUEST TO FIND THE ELIXIR:
Happiness Through 3-D Health

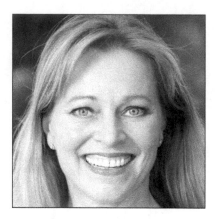

Eike Jordan

What on Earth is 3-D Health? It all started out in 2018. The Universe, or power of nature, decided that it is time for me to fulfill my duty and use my "powers," instead of neglecting, fearing, and hiding from them.

Since my childhood I had a variety of people, psychics, healers, and intuitives coming to me and insisting that I have 'magic' in me, and that I have guardian angels on my side who support my work. Patients state that my touch feels different—healing—as if my fingers have eyes.

My team calls me the galloping unicorn, the priestess, the empress, the heart of the universe. I love rainbows, nature, smelling the sweet blossoms, happy laughter, dancing, playing with my gumboots in the puddles (there is no bad weather, only the wrong clothes). I love happiness and BALANCE!

I always knew that there must be more. The addiction-like feeling of seeking more knowledge kept me looking into many areas of medicine, therapies, and the connection of art and science between body, mind, and soul—the heart of it all.

Let's look at some science and a few facts. Our pineal gland is situated right amongst the area of the brain that is responsible for emotions, feelings and eye/vision-function, melatonin production, and regulation of the wake-sleep cycle, the immune system, physical recovery, and healing. The mystery of endogenous DMT (N-Dimethyltryptamine) that is suspected to be produced by the pineal gland is only found these days in homeopathic amounts in the normal human body, and probably plays a major role. People state they experience deep happiness and lightness when being connected to the source under DMT influence. Is this the key to universal happiness and health, to seeing the whole, to access unlimited knowledge, and complete connection within?

Now what about melatonin, which is produced and regulated by the pineal gland? Melatonin inhibits dopamine release and may be present in regulation of addictive behavior. Are you aware that sugar is just as addictive as cocaine? Melatonin may correct behavioral disorders related to dopamine addiction and may ease cocaine/sugar withdrawal. The anti-excitatory effects of melatonin are even secondary to its incredible antioxidant effects. Further research in children shows that after administering melatonin in pharmacological doses, a reduction in severity and frequency of epileptic activity occurs.

Does the pineal gland release serotonin? To begin with, the pineal gland is located within the brain. Its main function is to release melatonin, which is released into the blood and possibly also into the brain fluid, known as cerebrospinal fluid. However, your train of thought isn't at all wrong; melatonin is purely derived from the chemical serotonin. Within the pineal gland serotonin is converted and utilized to produce melatonin.

Serotonin has a popular image as a contributor to feelings, happiness, and well-being. Its biological function is very multi-faceted and complex in modulating cognition, reward perception, learning, memory, and many other physiological processes. Serotonin is primarily found in the ENS (enteric nervous system) in the gastrointestinal tract, as well as it is produced in the CNS (central nervous system), located in the brain stem and stored in blood platelets. Ninety percent of the human body's total serotonin is produced in the gastrointestinal tract! There is a link between the lack of serotonin and depression. Serotonin is also a growth factor that plays a role in wound healing.

Suppressing emotions and feelings, substituting with drugs like sugars, Ayahuasca, etc. disables the area of the brain to produce endogenous DMT, melatonin, serotonin, and the ability to process data and to connect with the source. Negative, low frequency emotions imprint and reduce the ability to activate the pineal gland and important corresponding areas of the brain and body. Happiness and true love are the keys, disabling the EGO within, plus refusing sugars and other drugs to promote the production of endogenous hormones and support the healthy function of the entire endocrine system.

Brainwaves as overview:

	Brainwave Frequency	Body's Response	Aids in	Hormones / Neurotransmitters
Delta	0.5 – 4 Hz	Deep Rest / Sleep / Deep Meditation/ Subconscious learning	Sleep, Deepest Mediation	Melatonin, Human Growth Hormone
Theta	4 - 8 Hz	Deeply relaxed / Sleepy Feeling / REM stage of sleep, Inner Peace, Lucid Dreaming	Deep Meditation Insight, Creativity stimulates Immune System	Serotonin, GABA, Human Growth Hormone Endorphins, Anti-Cortisol, Acetylcholine
Alpha / Theta	7.83 Hz, Schumann Frequency	Physically Relaxed, Calm Sleepy, Meditative	Stimulates Immune System, decreased Insomnia EMF, Resistance	Endorphins, GABA, Serotonin, Acetylcholine
Low Beta	12.5 - 15 Hz	Power, Active, Busy, Anxious	Problem Solving, Active	GABA Dopamine

			Thinking, Data Processing	
Mid Beta	15 - 22 Hz	Active, Power Alert, Simulation of Pineal Gland	Focus Concentration Productivity Increase of IQ Stimulates Oxygen and Calcium Release	Dopamine
High Beta	22 - 38 Hz	Anxiety, Panic Attacks, Nervousness, Paranoia, Burn-out	Not helpful (ADD, ADHD)	Cortisol Adrenaline, Norepinephrine
Low Gamma	40 - 100 Hz	Feeling Oneness Ecstatic feeling REM stage sleep, during anaesthesia	Deep Meditation Enhanced Senses and peak performance, problem solving, heightened consciousness and perception	Disconnection Endorphins

How did I find the path to my breakthrough into happiness, health, and connecting with the highest levels of energy in the Universe? I learned at the tender age of seven years that the wrong nutrition leads to complete kidney failure despite all pharmaceuticals given. On top of the kidney failure, I looked like the hunchback of Notre Dame with severe scoliosis and wearing different heights of heels to compensate. Bless my parents for taking initiative and getting me every day of the week to either massage, physiotherapy, or chiropractic, and into swimming and other sports.

It was an incredible lesson to learn at such a young age!

The Universe directed my path to learn, on my own body, the various impacts of the good, the bad and the worst of habits and lifestyle. First and foremost, I learned to cut out all the sugars, including fruit, dairy, honey, as well as meat and shellfish. I put effort into preventative measures with a healthy, balanced diet, balanced physical activities, and regular therapies for my body. Just as I would maintain my vehicle (as my body IS my vehicle for life), and I kept studying and enhancing my left side brain.

- A balanced diet for my physical body enables healing and supports happiness.
- Various physical activities support brain health and happiness.
- Autogenic training and meditation enhance the brain's balance and performance and through that physical health and happiness.
- On and on it goes…

Now, none of the above is new to us. So why is it that the happiness and health doesn't last, and we still suffer no matter how hard we try? Why are there people living with the healthiest diet with a physically active lifestyle, yet they still get cancer or suffer a heart attack at age 45? And then there are those who live a super-unhealthy lifestyle; according to the books, they make it to unexpected old age but die after long suffering. Why is this?

The answer is the human factor. The EGO.

While I studied neurofeedback and biofeedback, I always achieved very high results on my brain capacity and performance. I first met Dr. Patrick Porter in the winter of 2017/2018 and tried his HRV and BrainTap technology. When I was tested by Dr. Porter's brother with the HRV, he found my brain performing at 76% capacity, whereas average result for Elite HRV users is 59.3%.

I love the BrainTap technology and started using it for myself, my family, and my patients. I became a big fan of Dr. Bruce Lipton's work about cellular behaviour and the subconscious. And I kept connecting the dots even further.

On March 17th, 2019, I had an accident while hiking with my puppies when I hit with my head hard on a sharp rock. I needed 11 stitches and it took three hours to stop the severe bleeding as nerves, muscles, and an artery were cut on my forehead. Additionally, I had a serious concussion, some sprains, strains, and a dislocated middle finger. It left a beautiful Harry Potter scar on my right eyebrow. This was a huge impact—but for good. When I was scanned with the HRV only two days after the incident, my brain performance despite the concussion was at an unbelievable 100%. That totally didn't make sense, but then again, it does.

While at the hospital and from then on, I felt deeply grateful for the care I received, the unconditional love I felt, and the support of everyone around me. I realized the EGO was in my way. I had to let go of me, my old beliefs, my limitations, increase empathy and feeling and embrace every bit of information that the Universe showers me with. The surprising outcome was that dropping my EGO increased my HRV results exponentially. I started to live in my heart and outside of my brain.

Now, everyone of us has a deep-rooted fear of negative emotion and imprint. Fair enough—we have the solution: adjust your belief system. Through 3-D Healing, you allow every negative imprint to be resolved and extracted right away. This allows us to open to positive, deep fulfilling happiness, love, and health.

The simple fact is that we exist on three levels of being: physical, emotional, and energetic. It requires all three levels to align and function for perfect health and happiness. A scar, a trauma, a dent, or a negative emotion in one or more of the levels sends ripples into the others and can, if ignored, cause chronic symptoms to various degrees.

Everything in the Universe has a frequency, a vibration. Even the Earth has the so-called Schumann Frequency measured in Hertz. Lately, this Earth vibration goes from a normal 7.83 Hz on the scale to high peaks of even up to 140 Hz. In scientific tests, animals and people showed being significantly impacted at around 30 Hz. Vibrating in happy alpha, low beta, delta and high gamma brain waves assists all of us to raise the flexibility within our cellular system.

Light has varying frequencies that display in a rainbow of colours. Some of us vibrate in blue, others are green, red, purple, yellow, orange, pink, and at the highest level, all these colours combine and turn into white, which resembles the highest frequency of vibration.

3-D health and healing means letting go of the EGO and working as a universal team, feeling empathy, evolving, and 'knowing', while practicing unconditional love. Our students and patients have said, "It feels like I had a non-invasive surgery in my body; I feel like I ran a marathon; I feel that the chains are taken away; I feel incredibly light and can actually breathe; I feel change is happening; I had no fear from the dentist anymore; I feel at peace; I am finally pregnant; I don't get angry anymore; my digestion functions; I no longer have migraines; my cysts are gone; I am happy and good things happen all of a sudden..."

Now you might be wondering, what is 3-D-healing?

The human body has many parts to it: the physical and the spiritual body, the peripheral nervous system, the right and left sides of the brain, Chakras—all of it guided and operated by the conscious and subconscious mind. All these parts of YOU are essential to YOUR health!

In 3-D Healing, we combine our medically trained therapists with the master level of spiritual therapists. Some of us reached the "Black Belt" master level in both departments. Working hand in hand as an open-minded team lets us achieve superior results with and for you.

3-D Healing is non-invasive. We don't want to know, nor do we need to know what is inside your head. We screen thoroughly for present and past injuries of your physical and emotional body. We recommend a thorough and very affordable assessment with HRV, NES, Darkfield blood microscopy, urine test, zinc tally test, and 119-point thermography. 3-D Healing comes with quality control in terms of always working as a team and regularly undergo the above tests ourselves!

Your body is 70% water. Just like water moves when you play music, thoughts and energies vibrate inside of you. 3-D Healing is your tool to open the gates and unblock stored negative emotions so their steady negative ripple effect can be removed, allowing healing to take place. During a light state of trance, your brain works within theta, alpha, and sometimes delta brainwaves. Within this very specific state of trance where you are in a heightened state of awareness, YOU can access your cellular system, DNA, and Higher Self to access the areas of trauma in order to get such information and negative energy ready for extraction (otherwise known as energetic surgery).

While in this very comfortable state, the 3-D team guides you safely along to the negative, unpleasant, fearful, and traumatic moments of life. Whether it is anxieties and deep-rooted fears, possible past lives, or energies that are not your own, we simply assist in releasing and resolving these inhibiting energies. You don't have to relive any of the experiences. The healthy frequencies of happiness are reinstated and enforced. Channeled quantum field energy transforms the body's frequencies, stimulating biochemical processes, and support healing mechanisms by unleashing the cellular intelligence of the human system, restoring the balance and connection to our center—the heart.

Our highly educated professionals access your body with your permission on non-physical energetic levels while you are in this light state of trance. Here, we recognize, find, and initiate healing in tissues, alignment of muscles and structures, speed up detoxification, and accelerate restoration, and reconnect chakras throughout the body for healthy flow of energy. Nutritional guidance and constitutional supplements are essential, as the health of both the physical and energetic body need to be equally supported for complete happiness and functionality.

For some people, all it takes is one session or even just meeting the team and being uplifted. Others it takes a few more sessions to get to the essence of happiness and the beauty of well-being, feeling love and compassion, to allow their brain to be in their heart, and to heal the heart.

Miracles are real, and they do happen—for me, for you, and for all of us!

Who can be part of 3-D Healing? Everybody that wishes to raise their levels of frequencies and is ready to let go of the EGO, and instead to connect back with the essence of deep love. From there, we can share the experience and knowledge and assist others to be lifted.

The most important part I learned is that we need all parts of the knowledge and wisdom that is out there—the modern medicine and pharmacy, traditional and ancient healing, energy, and spiritual and emotional healing. Everything functions synergistically, and the key is to know how to connect the modalities for the perfect outcome by acting as a team. To enable the pain-free breakdown of the walls, the barriers, the curtains within us, ultimately the fast and direct tool is 3-D Healing. We heal, repair, align, and balance the heart, brain, and system all throughout. Everyone can join the team and learn! You will find it uplifting.

Being the rainbow, overlapping and focussing colours to raise frequencies to the highest level, quality control as a team by the team, releasing the EGO, bringing feelings, gratefulness, openness, erasing judgement, and creating balance allows us, ALL TOGETHER, to BE the ELIXIR of Happiness and Health.

I am very passionate about health and happiness. We want to live longer, not die longer. Finding the elixir, seeing the whole picture completed, simple and yet so beautiful, this is pure joy! At the end of the day, it is about simplicity beyond complexity. We don't know what we don't know, but we can all learn.

Happiness, health and well-being is right inside us and available for each and everyone of us!

About the Author

Eike Jordan

Born 1968 in Hameln, and raised in Germany near Hannover, I came in 2006 to Canada and fell immediately in love with Vancouver Island.

I had my entire life long a great passion for healing, which was initiated by my own health problems as a child. I suffered from such serious nephritis that I was scheduled for dialysis and only then my parents decided to try a "witch doctor," which was back then the highly reputable Dr. Med. Bruker (1909-2001). He instantly changed my nutrition and switched to alternative medicine and homeopathy and saved my life. My kidneys regained, and maintained, to date full function. Further, I suffered from severe scoliosis and through the great teamwork of massage, physio, and chiropractic professionals, my spine turned into an upright, high performance part of my body and I was able to become a competitive athlete.

Parental genetics aren't the best in our family, and I decided to break the streak of that imprint by actively changing not only my nutrition and physical activities but as well in researching, learning and applying methods of healing to my own body to proof their beneficial effects.

Health and happiness are my passions – this has been my greatest desire my entire life long.

I love studying and researching, and I find that there is simply no limit to learning. I completely understand my colleagues and patients stating that it is difficult to find the time and financial resources to be able to get a chance to look into all the various areas of our being.

After finishing high school, I decided to first study in Germany Massage, Balneo-, Electro-, and Low-Intensity Laser Therapy, Foot Reflexology, Medical Foot Care (now Podiatry). I became manager of Physiotherapy in our Rehab Hospital, and added specialties to my repertoire such as Rheumatology, Respiratory Therapy, Permanent Disabilities. Plant based therapies (Phyto Chemistry is so fascinating), homeopathy, constitutional medicine, Iridology, Biofeedback, Neurofeedback, Darkfield Microscopy, and Clinical Hypnotherapy, Hyperthermia Therapy, Oxygen and Ozone Therapy, Cryotherapy, Redcord Neurac, Nutrition Counselling, Esthetic Lasers, and Microcurrent Therapy are just some of my many studies and certificates.

The key essential is I found out that our human body has many different layers and parts. The three main components are our physical, emotional, and our energetic body. If any of the three are in imbalance it affects the other part as well.

Detlef Joe Friede and I feel very blessed as co-founders to have found an incredibly effective way and approach to healing within every dimension: we named it 3-D Healing.

Contact Information:
Naturally Healthy Clinic
210 Milton Street
Nanaimo, BC, V9R 2K6
Canada
Phone +1.250.755.4051
Website: www.naturallyhealthyclinic.ca
Email: eike.jordan@n-h-clinic.com

RIVERS OF THOUGHT AND WHY IT SEEMS SO HARD TO CHANGE A THOUGHT

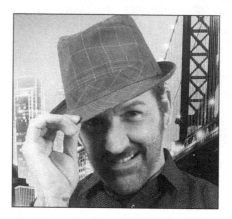

Kelly Fisher

My name is Kelly Fisher (K-FISH), and I have been a certified clinical hypnotherapist for over 23 years. While studying the mind and how it works, the conscious mind is 10 to 12% of your thought process, while the subconscious mind consists of 88 to 90% of your total thought process. You naturally have to study the brain and how that interplays with your mind and total thought process.

I like to separate the mind from the brain in this way.

The mind is the metaphysical study of how thoughts come to you conceptually. Most people do not have the capacity or knowledge of thinking original thoughts. That is why most people feel that their thoughts are thinking them. I have a process I teach called "L-Shape" Technique, where I teach clients to get into a meditative centered place where they can bring down original thought—maybe for the first time in their lives.

Without original thought, I call that your roof chatter, monkey mind, or little yip-yip dog that's trying to get your attention constantly. That part of your thinking is your conscious mind that you're reading this chapter right now. Unfortunately, most people think that roof chatter is who they are. They really believe the thoughts they think is who they are.

You don't have to believe everything you think. As a matter of fact, that is the best part of getting into a meditative practice. You have the ability to sit back and choose which thoughts you want to entertain and follow. It's a very powerful place to be!

Now for the brain. Every time you have a thought, your brain fires a chemical. This is what I call *rivers of thought*. As your brain fires this chemical, you feel the thought process. As a matter of fact, this firing process happens so fast and seemingly simultaneously that you can argue that thought-feeling is one action. For the purpose of this course of study, we will differentiate the two for educational purposes, because in truth they are on two different vibrational planes of existence even though experienced as one process.

This is the main reason it seems so hard to change your thoughts. The rivers of thought that you have been thinking for so many years becomes a part of your personality. In my live seminars I ask the audience, "If I had a magic wand and waved it across the room and took away all of your problems instantly, who would you be?"

Oh boy, does that get them thinking! They look up to the left, which is past. Then they look up to the right, which is future, and they can't find an answer to this question. This is because most people are so identified with their thoughts and problems that they think that's who they are. No one has ever given them the permission to dream properly.

So in short, your beliefs are just thoughts that you keep thinking. That seems so oversimplified to most people that they say, "Oh I just change my thoughts and my beliefs and my whole life will change?" YES! It is simple in concept but difficult in application, because your rivers of thought that you have been thinking your entire life has a chemical neural net that constantly fires up to such a degree that it just seems logical for you to think that way.

It takes some work to retrain your mind (your thought process), which then in turn retrains your brain to fire new chemicals of the neural net in a whole new way of thinking and feeling. But once you truly understand this is the ONLY way real change in your life takes place, you will not fight for your limitations.

Thought - Feeling - Emotion

Now we take it one step beyond the thought-feeling process that your mind and brain connect with and add in the physical emotion part of the equation. The emotion part of this equation is where we feel it out through the body or emote it out. Think of emotion as energy in motion!

The most important part where this Thought-Feeling-Emotion system comes into play is the longer you've been thinking, feeling, and emoting your thoughts out, the better chance it becomes a loop in your life. This means you're not sure if it's your emotions or your feelings or your thoughts that are controlling your life. You start to question and become confused about where you are actually stuck in your life. This is a legitimate question. The more important question to ask is "How do I stop this cycle?" Here is where you should always start.

In one of my main courses that I teach called "Anxiety Solution." Most of the time, especially if you've been thinking and feeling this way for a long time, it is much easier to break the physical, emotional part of your out of control thinking. This is where I start with all of my clients. If you took three breaths in as deep as you can and held them for as long as you can, you would break this anxiety circle and get back in control of your thoughts. I will have live links to my free training on ending anxiety in your life for good at the end of this chapter.

Free Training:

Beginners Meditation Guide to Ending Anxiety mp3

3 Things to Avoid when Ending Anxiety pdf

3 Part Video Workshop to "Control - Reduce - End" Anxiety in your Life — www.BestAnxietySolution.com

There are two basic different ways of thinking, feeling and emoting. Now, everything is by degree of course. That being said, you have your *high emos*, meaning high emotional people, and you have your *high physicals*. I am a high emo, meaning I think everything first and then say it out loud, if at all. My wife on the other hand is a high physical; she says everything out loud then thinks about it. Neither one is better than the other; it's just how we're hard wired.

A quick side note on relationships: we seek out the opposite of who we are (emos and physicals). This is what people mean when they say that opposites attract. It is also interesting to know when we do meet the opposite of who we are we try to act more like them, it's because we are attracted to them and want to make a good first impression. So when people say that you've fallen out of the "honeymoon" stage, what they are really saying is you've just fallen back into your natural being (emo-physical). Knowing this could save a lot of relationships.

My wife needs to constantly hear how much I love and care about her (high physical). I, on the other hand, know that we are married, have the same last name, and have a two-year-old child together. I am a high emo! It's just how we're hardwired.

I teach full courses on this Thought-Feeling-Emotion process.

Disconnecting from Thought-Feeling-Emotion

This is a HUGE, HUGE, HUGE, DISCLAIMER THAT I AM NOT A MEDICAL DOCTOR NOR HAVE I EVER SUGGESTED TO ANYONE TO STOP THEIR PRESCRIBED MEDICATION OR TO EVEN CHANGE OR ALTER THEIR PRESCRIBED MEDICATION TREATMENT BY THEIR DOCTORS IN ANY WAY!

I say this in print this way because in my private hypnotherapy practice, I tell my clients this information I'm about to tell you.

You have to understand that when you introduce a chemical into your system to "make you feel better," this chemical does not do that—it makes you not feel at all. Please know that I'm not trying to alter your viewpoint on what your doctor says. But the clients that I've been working with over the last 23 years all say the same thing to me. What they share is after taking this prescribed medication from their doctor, "I don't feel at all." This is true because when you take a prescribed medication from your doctor, it cuts off one of the three levels of Thought-Feeling-Emotion that we are all born with.

It is very important to know that you don't feel better; you don't feel at all. Now I know from my private practice if you're going through mental HELL with your own thoughts, feeling NOTHING is far better than feeling this hell that you are going through. Thus, you naturally think that this prescribed medication is working. I'm telling you from my decades of experience, this temporary relief you are feeling is NOT the way to permanently change your thought process in a positive way that you are looking for. Once you take this chemical mask off, you will have to deal with your personal problems right where you left off when you started to mask them.

Everybody that knows how the mind works knows that this information is true. But they are scared of being sued. I just feel someone has to say this out loud. Like I said, I explain this to all of my clients because I truly want the best and quickest way to my clients to get back in control of their thought process so they can truly change, get in control, and make the permanent changes in their lives that they're looking for!

I will reiterate for the fact I AM NOT A MEDICAL DOCTOR NOR HAVE I EVER SUGGESTED TO ANYONE TO STOP THEIR PRESCRIBED MEDICATION OR TO EVEN CHANGE OR ALTER THEIR PRESCRIBED MEDICATION TREATMENT BY THEIR DOCTORS IN ANY WAY!

Quickest Way to Reprogram Your Brain and Why We Meditate

In this part of the teaching, I want to explain to you what I call "The Full Glass Syndrome/Emotional Overspill" theory. Visualize a glass of water filled all the way to the top. Now every time you had to deal with anything, this full glass syndrome would tilt over to the slightest degree and you would have an emotional overspill.

I have been blamed for having no emotional reaction and therefore not in touch with my emotions. The truth is I am in such control over my thoughts and what feelings I chose to feel that I don't just emote everything out. Plus remember, I'm a high emo! So when most people say, "Oh, he or she's so emotional," what they're really saying is that person is emotionally out of control. You don't want to be that person.

The main reason we practice meditation is during meditation sessions we lower that full glass syndrome to let's say half full. Afterward, each and every time you have a problem in your life, you now have the capacity to deal with these new problems in a very different way than before, thus in control of your Thoughts-Feelings-Emotions. This is a beautiful way to live. I have whole video teaching this "Full Glass Syndrome/Emotional Overspill" concept at https://vimeo.com/171457619/c8d40f6d1c

Just so you understand, this woo-woo concept is really not a woo-woo concept at all. It's funny because I just had this conversation today about the things that I study are so woo-woo. I think that most people (like you) are coming around to the fact that these woo-woo concepts are actually the way all people think and feel, and this is the true path to getting in control of your thoughts, feelings, and emotions that most people are looking for.

Tying It All Together (What do you really want out of life?)

The truly happy brain completely responds to your thoughts first, then simultaneously fires a chemical neural net like a river carving into the hardest of rock. Yes, the grey matter moves with neuroplasticity and expands with greater flexibility. Not all analogies are perfect, but that's why I call it "Rivers of Thought," because the more you think a certain thought a certain way, the easier it is to fire up and keep thinking that thought as truth.

This is why it seems so hard to change a thought. With a little practice and positive mental gymnastics, you can think whatever thought you want at any time you want to right on the spot. That is the true meaning of responsibility, meaning your ability to respond to any situation at any given time.

Remember, there are many definitions that relate to the mind and the brain, like "The mind is a horrible master, but the mind is an excellent servant." That can go along with the brain as well.

I still meditate twice a day to re-center myself and to get so much more accomplished in a shorter time than if I just tried to muscle through my day. The muscling approach will definitely burn anyone out. How many people do you know that are overwhelmed and completely burned out on life? This is why! Meditating every day will soon be just like brushing your teeth every day. I exercise every day, sometimes twice a day, because I just know the benefits and the amazing feelings I get from taking care of me first. If that statement sounds selfish or self-centered to you, then you have to think of the analogy of being on an airplane with your young child and the oxygen masks fall down. The flight attendants always say to put your oxygen mask on first, then save your child. If you're not taking care of yourself first, then you really have nothing left to give to anyone else.

Make your brain happy with meditation every day and exercise to feed that happy brain with fresh oxygen. What you're going to get out of life is exactly going to match your effort you put in. This includes meditation, exercise, and overall positive thinking in any given situation. It's like when people say to me, "Oh I tried meditation once. That didn't work for me." No, it worked exactly to the degree of effort that you put into it. Just like if you said, "I've tried exercise once, and that didn't do anything for me." No, you burned the exact number of calories for the effort you put into it.

Don't judge your overall goals to whether or not you've achieved them by the smallest of effort. These things accumulate, compound, and have an expanded quickening to get to your goals even faster.

In short, never ever give up. We don't have that much time on this vibrational plane of Maya. (At least this incarnation.)

My special Free Gift to you for purchasing this book and reading my chapter: I am discounting 50% off my six-week online course, "Anxiety Solution: Slow Your Mind Down to the Speed You're Living" at www.BestAnxietySolution.com/anxiety. On the checkout page enter code: GET50PERCENTOFF

About the Author

Kelly Fisher

Kelly is a certified clinical hypnotherapist and certified life coach. In his practice of helping people, he automatically sees vision far beyond what they can see for their own life. Whether in the office or during Skype sessions all across the country, Kelly and his clients go through the hypnotherapy part of the session. He literally fills the room with energy and shows them how to plug back into their own source of energy, so they leave his office and Skype Session every time feeling far, far better than when they came started. He feels blessed to professionally study this subject. He is also blessed not only to be awake his whole entire life but blessed to have a career that he can hand down and teach other people how to wake up, plug in, and know that they are their own loving energy source and don't need anything else other than that.

Kelly has been studying his whole life on how the mind and brain works, of how we think, and why we feel and how to interpret on all six levels of our perception. Reach out to him so you can jump to the front of the line on this deep metaphysical understanding and have a very, very dramatic life-changing experience.

Kelly also has an amazing six-week in-depth online training program called "Anxiety Solution: Slow Your Mind Down to the Speed You're Living."
www.BestAnxietySolution.com
www.BestAnxietySolution.com/anxiety

Fall Asleep Instantly Free pdf
www.FallAsleepInstantly.com

He helps women heal from infidelity without guilt or blame so they can be whole again.
"H.A.R.R.P.: 5 Stages of Infidelity"
www.StagesofInfidelity.com

To get a copy of his current book, Weight loss from the Inside Out: A Mind and Body Awakening, and his groundbreaking guided visualization audio program, Weight Loss Through Hypnosis, reach out to him at www.GlobalMindStretch.com

Contact Information:
Email: GlobalMindStretch@gmail.com

WAKE UP!
Get to the *HEART* of the Matter and Let Your Spirit Soar

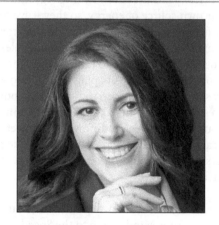

Michelle Dion
Board Certified Naturopathic Doctor

"Above all else, guard your heart,
for everything you do flows from it."

- Proverbs 4:23

A book about healthy brains would not be complete without a chapter devoted to our heart-brain connection and the emerging new field known as *neurocardiology*. The expression "getting to the heart of the matter" or the "crux of the matter" stems from the Latin meaning of crux, meaning "cross." In English, it means "difficulty" or "puzzle," and heart is meant as a "vital part." Our heart is referred to as our intrinsic cardiac nervous system or "little brain." It is the central hub of intelligence for our intuitive regulation of emotional experiences. How we handle our emotions has a direct effect on our mental and physical well-being. It also plays a role in our connections with our true essence of spirit and can either move us closer to or further away from enlightenment.

Emotional intelligence is defined as "our capacity to be aware of, control, and express one's emotions, and to handle interpersonal relationships judiciously and empathetically. It is the key to both personal and professional success." The more we have the skills to self-regulate, the better we are able to communicate effectively, reduce stress and the toll it takes on our bodies in its role in disease, diffuse conflicts, improve relationships, empathize with others, and effectively overcome life's challenges to be able to share our true spiritual gifts with the world and manifest our wishes, hopes, and dreams. It is the difference between our ability to not only survive, but also to thrive.

In his book, *Power Vs. Force*, David Hawkins takes a look at the power that comes from within as we are able to navigate the map of consciousness to operate in higher levels of positive emotional vibration. The scale ranges from 0 with emotions like shame and guilt up to a level of 1,000, where enlightenment is. Emotions below 200 are destructive of life in the individual and society at large. All values above 200 are where our constructive expression of our power lies. Courage is the tipping point right at 200.

Isn't that interesting? Human nature resists change and in order to take steps out of our comfort zone, we must first learn to walk in courage. It's important to understand that emotions are not good or bad per se; they are all part of life and important signals that give us clues when we are out of harmony and alignment with something. Once we get the message, we want to use it to take action and not allow the situation to keep us stuck at the lower levels of destruction.

Awakening to the wisdom of our heart's intelligence is the key to unlocking the door to a higher level of consciousness to make manifest the glory of God that is within each of us. Discovering our soul's true purpose comes from the transformation we are invited to allow to unfold through life's rollercoaster of emotional ups and downs and trials and tribulations, or what I would call defining moments.

Defining moments are snapshots of time in life that can threaten to shake us at the core of our being. Some are exhilarating moments of happiness, sheer joy, ecstasy, rapture, calmness, and peacefulness. Others are at the other end of the spectrum like sadness, grief, shock, fear, anger, anxiety, hopelessness, and despair. They all have purpose and meaning and form the rich tapestry of our lives and create the stories we tell ourselves and choose to believe. These are memories that we catalog in a file cabinet in our brains, and emotions we feel and store in the recesses of our hearts. We can either choose to allow these moments to define us or transform us. It is in these circumstances that we are given an opportunity to step up our level of consciousness and self-mastery both individually and collectively. It is a time where we can either choose to awaken to the power within and allow a new awareness to propel us forward and upward or we can choose to stay stuck and accept the status quo.

I invite you to ponder with me the current *pulse* of humanity and our interconnectedness to one another as a community. We are all spiritual beings having human experiences, traveling along the road of life. We are each unique in our own way yet share many common threads. Just like a snowflake, no two people are exactly alike. One snowflake by itself is not nearly as impressive or powerful as a beautiful winter wonderland landscape where it takes millions of snowflakes to come together to create such a masterpiece. Never underestimate your worth or your ability to make a difference when you align with others to raise consciousness. It is your divine right to shine your light brightly and to live a life of abundance. This is not just for some of us; it is meant for all of us. We are each a microcosm within a macrocosm, and each of us do indeed matter. We are called to be a mirror for one another, to serve, encourage, uplift, and hold space for each other's growth.

As a collective, we have certainly experienced some defining moments. When you ask people what they were doing when they got news the first man walked on the moon, JFK was shot, or the Twin Towers went down, most people can remember and describe those moments vividly and in great detail. These are examples of such collective moments we have experienced individually yet those we have also shared as a community and as a nation.

I think that sometimes we forget that we all began our life in the same way and are therefore created equal. When we develop in our mother's womb, our heart tube begins beating spontaneously independent of any other stimulus in the first trimester. This initial beating happens before our heart is fully formed into chambers, and our neural tube has completed the formation of the different areas of our brain and brain stem. When we are further along in development, our heart and brain begin to sync and establish a communication highway back and forth. The constant chatter/conversation that goes on between our heart brain and our head brains are predominantly afferent. This means that our heart sends more information up to the brain than the brain sends down to the heart.

As our heart is beating, the space between each heartbeat creates a rhythm. This rhythm produced by our heart is the most powerful rhythm in our bodies. Our brain, digestion, and respiratory systems all respond to this rhythm. The rhythm can either be chaotic or coherent, and we can use a tool known as HRV, or heart rate variability, to measure this rhythm. The rhythm reflects the natural changes that occur in between heartbeats. Over a short period of time, we can see the pattern that is created that reflects our heart-brain communication and the dynamics of our nervous system in response to positive and negative emotions. When we experience negative emotions like anger, anxiety, grief, or sadness, it produces chaotic rhythms and when we experience positive emotions like joy, peace, happiness, and love, it produces more coherent rhythms. We are either in a state of energy expenditure or energy renewal.

Coherence implies that the parts of a whole are in alignment together and working harmoniously. In our own bodies, coherence happens when our heart, mind, nervous system, and spirit become synchronized. This is much like the different tones of the various singers' voices in a choir or different instruments in an orchestra coming together in harmony to produce a beautiful melody or song. Coherence creates better energy efficiency and allows us to make better decisions. It is a higher physiological state than just relaxation. When we are coherent, we put our bodies in a state most conducive for optimal healing as it can renew our energy and give us the reset we need, such as before standing up and giving a presentation, after a difficult and upsetting interaction, to heal from an illness, or to make important decisions.

We can use tools to help us practice coherence such as the tools and techniques we employ the use of in my office from the HeartMath Institute as well as others. Much like practicing to improve sport performance, intentionally practicing these techniques can help us build resilience to navigate the ups and downs of life more efficiently and effectively. Every single one of us faces stressors, both the internal ones we create within ourselves and the external ones that come at us from the outside world. When we have better resilience, we are more equipped and ready to handle challenges.

The mere definition of resilience is "the capacity to adapt from and recover quickly from difficulties; toughness." Like an elastic band, it can be stretched yet springs back to form. "In the study of Physics, the power or ability to return to the original form or position after being bent, compressed, or stretched; elasticity." Building up coherence is like building a nest egg of savings in a bank account. If enough reserves are built up in there, we have a supply for those blindsiding moments of incidental expenditures. If we don't, when the rubber band is stretched beyond limitations, it snaps.

Emotions are nothing more than energy in motion. Nikola Tesla said, "If you want to find the secrets of the universe think in terms of energy, frequency, and vibration." Our heart generates the largest electromagnetic field in the body. This field is measured by an electrocardiogram and is about 60 times greater than the brain waves in amplitude recorded by an EEG. HeartMath studies show this field can be detected and measured several feet away from the person's body and between others within a close proximity. Can you think about a time when you may have picked up on the energy of another? You know, those times you walk in the room and feel like you could cut the tension with a knife? Or how about when someone really happy and energetic walks in and suddenly brightens up the entire room? Both negative emotions and positive emotions can be perceived and felt by others.

Let me give you an example of an incident in my life so that you may draw examples from your own. My earliest memory is from when I was two years old. I can remember everything about it like it was yesterday. From my maternal grandparent's living room, I witnessed my great-grandmother having a fatal heart attack. I took everything about the experience in through my senses. From seeing the sweat pour down her face and over her body, to the smell of her vomit, to the sound of the ambulance coming up the driveway, to my grandmother's shaking touch as she sat me down in my rocking chair, asking me to stay seated while the paramedics rushed by us to work on her. It was all very surreal.

As I sit here writing this, I can actually feel my body start to rock as if I am in that rocking chair now, trying to self-soothe and feeling a sense of terror in my body that is sending signals to flood cortisol through my veins. This is the fight or flight reaction we have all experienced from time to time when our bodies perceive threats, whether they are physical or emotional in nature. At two years old, our cortex (the thinking rational brain) is not yet fully developed. Although I didn't have the capacity at that age to totally understand and process what was happening logically, I did feel the emotions of everyone in that room energetically.

That incident was 48 years ago, yet I can still experience it as if it were happening at this exact moment in time when I intentionally think about it. You see, our bodies store these incidents and traumas. I cataloged the incident in the file cabinet in my brain and in my heart. These incidents can be reactivated through a similar trigger to one of those five senses or just the mere thought of it or an emotion towards it. This is much like what happens for people dealing with PTSD. For a long time, until I became aware and did some work on changing my brain's neuroplasticity from this incident, I was triggered by sweating. I would also get anxiety seeing, hearing, or smelling someone's vomit, or any time I would see or hear any type of flashing lights.

Much like we leave the frequency/energy/DNA of our fingerprints on a glass we drink out of long after we leave a room or building, our stored thoughts and emotions leave imprints in the cells of our bodies and in our energetic fields long after they occur. These broadcast messages like radio waves. Every time we replay the same thought or emotion, the neuroplasticity in our brain becomes stronger. This is true of both positive and negative signals. Like begets like, so it is important to pay attention to the signals we consciously and unconsciously generate.

Sometimes we can get stuck in an endless loop tape between our negative emotions and our negative thoughts; one seems to keep feeding the other in a vicious cycle. It's this spiral that can send us further down into our deep, dark abyss and keep us from healing or achieving our goals and manifesting our desires. It is not just our surface conscious thoughts, but it includes all those background noise messages from our subconscious. Positive affirmations are not enough to shift us because although we may say or think something, if we don't align that thought with a positive feeling of belief, we are not truly broadcasting that message to manifest it. We must also get into the emotion of the affirmation. Act as if and feel as if it has already happened.

Let's take a moment to get into coherence now. One of the easiest ways to shift a negative thought or feeling is to get into a state of gratitude. "In everything give thanks and praise; for this is God's will for you in Christ Jesus" (1 Thessalonians 5:18). What if instead of moaning about our circumstance or rehashing it, we were to express and have a grateful or contrite heart? What if we were to look upon our hard time as an opportunity to grow and climb the ladder to enlightenment and higher consciousness? Just like I recounted a situation when I could remember negative emotions coursing through my body, I would ask you now to think about a time you felt sincere appreciation and gratitude for someone or something and notice what shifts you feel in your body.

Now, focus on the area of your heart. Imagine as you breathe that a beautiful vibrant white light is emanating from your chest. Breathe in and out a little slower and a little deeper. If it helps, you can count your breaths in rhythmic fashion. For example, breathe into a count of five and out to a count of five. Now, bring in that feeling of gratitude or appreciation as you continue your breathing pattern. Wash that feeling over and throughout your body and then imagine the light carrying outside of you to others. Try to stay in that feeling intentionally for as long as you can. If you mind starts to wander, just bring your attention back to the area of the heart and feel your heart beating. You can repeat this any time throughout the day.

Whether we find ourselves on a journey back to optimal health and wellness from a state of "dis – ease," experience the stress of a toxic relationship, are worried about the state of our financial situation, feel pressure from a deadline, or have endured some trauma, getting to the heart of the matter in learning to regulate our energetic fields of vibration is the key to changing the situation and manifesting something different. Illness, injury, and trauma can all serve as opportunities for us to wake up to higher levels of consciousness to make manifest the glory of God that is within each of us. As spiritual beings having human experiences, we all must choose whether we will let these life lessons define or transform us. The choice is ours and ours alone. We were each given the gift of free will. To whom much is given, much is required. What comes along with our gift of this freedom of choice is the responsibility that those choices have direct cause-and-effect outcomes or consequences on ourselves and those around us.

When we choose to get to the heart of the matter and take responsibility for our choices and well-being, our spirits can soar. We can contribute our unique gifts to our families and communities. Not only do we vibrate at a higher frequency, but we also help lift up and elevate others. Just like science is now learning that trees link roots underground, sending nutrients and communicating with each other, it's vitally important that we join in community to collectively vibrate at higher levels of consciousness. I invite you and hope to see you at a Global Coherence hotspot soon.

I will close with a quote from one of my mentors, Dr. David J. Pesek:

"When love and wisdom unite, expect a masterpiece."

About the Author

Michelle Dion

Michelle Dion is a naturopathic doctor and is board certified through the American Naturopathic Medical Certification Board. She is a certified holistic nutrition consultant and holds a diplomate in holistic iridology. Additionally, Michelle is a Health Rhythms facilitator and a certified HearthMath instructor.

Michelle owns and operates A Call to Spirit, LLC, a holistic wellness education center located in Chantilly, Virginia. She has completed her certification for A Call to Spirit to be a Global Coherence Hotspot to gather community members to help raise global consciousness. She enjoys successful collaboration amongst other professionals in the healthcare industry and is a founding member of the Northern Virginia Group of Metro Collaborative. Michelle is also an independent certified coach, speaker, and trainer with The John Maxwell Team.

Contact Information:
A Call to Spirit, LLC
Email: acalltospirit@aol.com
Website: www.acalltospirit.com
          www.johnmaxwellgroup.com/MichelleDion
          www.metrocollaborative.com/members/michelle-dion
Telephone: 703-955-7055

PEMF FOR A HAPPY BRAIN

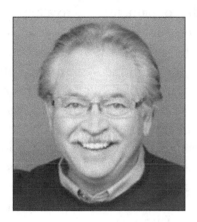

Pat Ziemer

In this chapter, I will provide you with an overview of PEMF and how Magna Wave PEMF utilizes this therapy for human health and wellness. Inflammation is the number one cause of pain in the body. The use of Pulsed Electromagnetic Fields (PEMF) provides a means to reduce inflammation, thereby reducing and relieving pain. The primary function is to improve oxygenation and blood flow in the body.

Magnetic fields affect the charge of the cell membrane, which opens up the cells' membrane channels. These channels are like the doors and windows of a house for airflow and circulation. By opening cell channels, nutrients are easily absorbed by the cell and waste is easily eliminated. The process helps to rebalance and restore optimum cell function. If you utilize PEMF to restore cells continually, they will work more efficiently. By using PEMF for restoring or maintaining cellular function, you will in turn repair or maintain organ function, allowing the entire body to function better and maintain wellness.

We also know that the body ages over time, and that an

essential part of slowing the aging process is to keep the function of every individual cell at an optimal level. A byproduct of this cellular rejuvenation process provided by Magna Wave PEMF is the feeling of wellbeing that occurs when optimum cellular health is maintained. This process of optimum cellular health becomes the basis for excellent results for many indications by providing the relief of pain, leading to a happy brain.

A new angle on Alzheimer's, depression, anxiety, stroke, and concussions is the inflammation connection. Recent studies have shown how the immune system and inflammation play a role in the development of these conditions and how targeting specific elements of the inflammatory process could be useful in treating or preventing these and other disorders. Various drugs and medications are given to fight the body's inflammation processes. The use of Magna Wave PEMF has demonstrated the promise of a drug-free method of fighting the damaging effects of inflammation as a part of the disease process. The PEMF modality has gained FDA clearance for uses that include non-union fractures, depression, autism, incontinence, and brain tumors. The PEMF modality is used regularly to improve any indication that could benefit from improved oxygenation and inflammation reduction. The list of positive results is long and growing, including everything from arthritis to stress-related diseases and by often providing a speedier recovery.

The incidence of concussions and traumatic brain injuries (TBIs) represent a rising concern in the area of sports, military activities, and work injuries. As reported in the *Journal of Neurology* (Brain 2019: 142255-262), there is a scientifically proven method for measuring brain voltage using a combination of a quantitative electroencephalogram (QEEG), coupled with a test known as the P300 (Evoked Potential). The available research shows that brain voltage typically drops following a concussion and is the last physiological measurement to return to a healthy state following a head injury.

Quite often, the only medical advice given to the post-concussion patient is to rest. However, there might be other mechanisms by which an individual can recover more efficiently while reducing the risk of future concussions. Magna Wave is currently working with Dr. Larry Lyons, a psychologist in San Diego, California, researching the use of high-powered PEMF to increase brain voltage and improve brainpower or neural output. The brain and body will "mimic" the PEMF fed into it, and capillary blood flow will increase. Inflammation can limit the success of other types of biofeedback; PEMF can reduce inflammation while administered at fast speeds without generating heat and damaging tissue. PEMF can also be used to entrain the brain via operant conditioning or dis-entrain the brain via de-habituation. It has been hypothesized that in the brain, PEMF increases nitric oxide, which induces vasodilation, enhances microvascular perfusion and tissue oxygenation, and may be a useful adjunct therapy in traumatic brain injury.

In the present San Diego study, participants will undergo a quantitative electroencephalogram (QEEG) to obtain a baseline measure of their brain voltage. Participants will then receive a total of six PEMF sessions over three weeks using the Magna Wave system. For treatment, the coils will be placed on the temporal regions of the brain. The participants will then be retested with the QEEG to determine brain voltage (i.e., how many neurons fire in unison when novel stimuli is presented in the P300 auditory task), and brain speed changes (how fast it takes the brain to recognize a change in stimuli). By examining brain speed with brain voltage, an approximate brain age can be calculated. By breaking down the test results to the phrase "Brain age," it becomes an easy reference point for a person to comprehend. It will be interesting to see if high-powered PEMF as administered by the Magna Wave technology can create a more youthful brain. The formula is presented below:

BRAIN SPEED (in milliseconds) x BRAIN POWER (voltage) = BRAIN AGE

CASE STUDIES

Stroke-related Aphasia

Aphasia is a condition that often occurs following a stroke. It is a condition where someone can no longer speak in sentences, or they struggle to find the words that they're trying to say. What follows is a case study on a client who suffered from severe aphasia as a result of a stroke.

Dale was treated for his aphasia for three years at a stroke rehabilitation center. He was released because they felt Dale had advanced as far as he could with their therapy processes. Dale's wife, a friend of my wife, asked if we could treat him to see if our process would provide additional improvement of his condition. Our response was an absolute yes, and we were excited to have the opportunity to improve Dale's life. We requested approval from the stroke rehabilitation center, and they said it was fine. We enlisted the help of a speech therapist to give us some direction on ways to work with him.

Dale began his daily visits to our office for a 15 to 20-minute treatment session. For his regular protocol, we would treat the area of injury and cognition area of the brain. We would switch up the attachments used between the butterfly loop, the paddle, and the large loop. Our basic protocol was treating for six minutes on the area of injury, six minutes on the area of cognition, and then another six to 10 minutes on the upper chest and upper back. The purpose was to improve proper blood oxygenation and blood flow throughout the body.

We began to treat Dale daily, and for the first two or three weeks, we didn't see anything happen. Dale was growing impatient because he was anxious to see it work. At one point, he tried to quit, but because we had developed a friendship, we persuaded him to continue with the process. Our protocol was to go through flashcards on his computer. We would show him a picture and ask him what it was, and then we would flip the screen and show the word. After three additional weeks of treatment, we began to see some improvement. He could recognize the pictures and say the words much more quickly and make a better association between words and pictures. When he first came to the office, Dale would always have a small notebook that he would use to point at words or write down what he was trying to say. Over time, he would use the notebook with less frequency because he was able to speak specific words to help move communication along.

At one point in his career, Dale was a concert promoter, and

I was a drummer in a rock band, so this allowed our collective interests to spur conversations. He had worked with Jimmy Buffett, so he would pull out his notebook and point to Jimmy Buffett's name to start a conversation, but it remained a struggle. As we pursued further PEMF sessions, he would come in and say, "Jimmy Buffet asked how we were doing," and on occasion he could make full sentences. He improved to the point that he was able to improve his speech and cognition by 35 to 40%. He and his family were able to resume some form of verbal communication that was almost totally lost previously. We continued the sessions daily for nearly a year, and he continued to see moderate improvement and was more comfortable in his conversations.

We got to the point that we told his wife that we felt that we had helped all that we could and that it was not necessarily for him to come daily for sessions. Her response was, "No, you can't quit," and we asked why. She said, "Because he is no longer depressed. He comes home smiling, he's happy, he wants to talk, and take walks. His depression is virtually gone, and we feel that it's a result of your Magna Wave PEMF treatments." So we continued our sessions and developed a deeper personal relationship with Dale.

Our conclusion was that the process helped him regain some speech and cognition. The PEMF sessions also enhanced his sense of wellbeing and helped to relieve his depression. We continued for another year to work with Dale, and he remained a very happy person. Dale passed away unexpectedly from other complications about a year later. We felt fortunate that we were able to use PEMF to provide Dale with a better quality of life and a happier brain as he dealt with life after his stroke.

Depression

Clinical, non-responsive depression is a condition where someone does not respond to conversational therapy, medication therapy, or electrotherapy. This is considered one of the more severe types of depression.

What follows is a case study of a client who I will call "Mary." She was referred to us by a friend because she suffered from severe depression and could no longer work. She was suicidal and would find herself at home, unable and not wanting to go anywhere or do anything. My friend asked me if our therapy could potentially help Mary. I answered yes and explained that studies had shown good results with depression. I encouraged him to have her come to the office and begin sessions so we could research and document her progression. I can say that when Mary came into the office, it was a pretty amazing sight. She came in wearing sweatpants and a sweatshirt, appearing disheveled. Mary wouldn't look upward. She frowned all the time and could hardly move securely.

We explained the therapy and told her what we hoped to accomplish. We told her that because it could take some time to begin to see results, we wanted to treat her daily. She understood and agreed, so we started our treatments. In addition to treating her head, neck, and shoulders, we did overall body treatments for her upper body and lower back. We also focused on her feet weekly to stimulate the reflexology points. After the initial two weeks, we didn't see any dramatic results, and she was very down and still depressed, ready to quit. We were able to convince her to continue the sessions for three weeks before stopping the process. By agreeing to stay with the program, it seemed that she opened the door for it to work because within two weeks when she would come in, she showed improvement.

Not as disheveled and more alert, she would come with a slight smile and began walking around the office and saying hello to everyone. As we continued the process, we treated her Monday through Friday for 15 or 20-minute sessions. She would regress over the weekend and we would have to play catch-up for a couple of days. Over time, it got to the point that she wouldn't regress as much over the weekend, but it would always backtrack if she did not continually receive treatment.

After six months of regular treatment, she was a different person. Mary was dressing normally, not afraid to be in public, and started talking about going back to work. After eight months, she decided that she wanted to have a machine that she could use at home to treat herself. She intended to treat herself only as needed to hopefully reduce the number of visits per week, and that's what happened. Mary progressed to the point that she managed herself only as necessary to support her wellbeing. She was able to make that transition after about a year of regular treatment.

My mantra is to continue treatment as long as function continues to improve and then as necessary to maintain improved service.

Mary wanted to work, and she started to work with us part-time. She began to talk about different jobs that would fit her renewed wellness. Her love was tourism, and she was able to find a job in travel planning that she had done prior to her debilitating depression. When this process began, Mary was on total disability and did not have a good future. The utilization of Magna Wave PEMF therapy helped bring her to where she was able to regain the life that she so much wanted to live. While the PEMF modality continues to grow and mature, there remains much to learn and explore with Pulsed Electro-Magnetic Field therapy. What I do know from 19 years of experience utilizing PEMF, whatever the condition is, the relief of pain leads to a happy brain.

About the Author

Pat Ziemer

Pat Ziemer is the owner of Magna Wave and has been working full-time with PEMF since 2002. The company's therapy devices are used extensively on racehorses, performance horses, and professional athletes. Seven recent Kentucky Derby winners and numerous world champions in many horse disciplines utilize this therapy regularly. In 2007, Pat acquired the rights to the PEMF device, repackaged it, branded it as Magna Wave, and hit the road, marketing the Magna Wave brand. Since 2007, the company has placed over 2,000 Magna Wave devices onto the market for private and professional use. Magna Wave now services human, small animal, and equine markets.

Contact Information:
Websites: www.PEMFprofessionals.com
www.MagnaWavePEMF.com

WHAT IF?

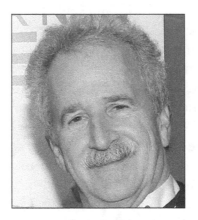

Stan Esecson

"What if?" Those two simple words might be the most powerful words in the English language. What if something as simple as changing your socks could instantly change your brain? Well, that's exactly what's been happening. We see it clinically in QEEG brain scans that have been analyzed by some of the top doctors in the world. These brain scans were done with a patient wearing their socks, eyes open, then retested eyes closed. The tests were repeated with the patient wearing our socks. To remove bias, some tests have been done with our socks first. These socks are literally poised to change the world! I know what you're thinking, "Socks?" but please keep reading.

Let me set the stage and tell you how I was introduced to this product. I'm an idea guy. I had never held a job in my life. Fortunately, I've had enough of the good ideas that have helped pay for some of the stupid ones, but you never know which was which in the beginning. Two years ago, my phone rang, and it was a buddy from Florida. He said he came across an amazing new product from Canada, and, "With your marketing mind, you'll be fascinated!" I told him I was quite happy, really busy, making plenty of money, and already getting up at 4:30 every morning. I had enough on my plate and just wasn't looking to add anything else to my life at the moment, so I said, "Thanks, but no thanks." He persisted and repeated, "You'll be fascinated." Well, now I was getting more irritated than fascinated, so I rudely barked, "What is it?" He responded, "It's a pair of socks." I just started laughing over the phone.

I said, "You've got to be kidding me! I'm not going to talk to people about socks." He replied, "You really owe it to yourself to check this out." He emailed me a couple of videos. I watched them and called him right back telling him, "Come on, it's just a magic trick." He said, "No, it's real. You'll see."

He then proceeded to make perhaps the best business decision of his life and overnighted me some socks and insoles (as both have the same technology). On Sundays I would take my 93-year-old mother out to lunch. I drove over and picked up my mom. We drove to the restaurant, I parked the car, opened her door, and she got out. I asked her to take off her shoes as I wanted to do a little experiment. Picture this: we're in a busy parking lot in Southern California, and I'm asking a great-grandmother to take off her shoes. Anyway, I say, "Mom, stand up straight, arms by your side. I'm going to stand next to you and gently try to tip you over, so try not to tip." I tried, and of course she tips. Next, I say, "Step on the insoles." She did that and I tried again but I could not budge her. This frail, 93-pound elderly woman instantly became stronger, more stable, and I could not tip her over.

That's when it clicked. My friend was right, and this was something very special. My mom wasn't trying to con me, she wasn't trying to sell me anything, and she had no clue what was happening. The bottom line was that she was stronger and more stable the moment she stood on these insoles. That's a big deal. If you know any older people, ask them. You'll discover that one of their biggest fears is the fear of falling and hitting their head or breaking a hip, either of which can be tragic.

Three days later, I hopped on a plane and flew to Toronto, as I wanted to meet the inventor, Jay. I wanted to look him in the eye and make sure that there was a real company behind this product because I saw the writing on the wall. I was going to help spread the word and get this product to millions of people. It was while meeting with Jay that I discovered his vision, his passion, the backstory, and his goal to get these socks on a billion feet.

Jay's mom was diagnosed with MS, and he watched her go from diagnosis to wheelchair in a matter of 18 months. He retired from the computer industry and made his new mission to help improve the quality of her life. He was convinced that her issue was neurological. He was equally convinced that there has been a lot of profound medical research done around the globe, but most of it was sitting in silos. Harvard did a study on this, Columbia did a study on that, Yale did a study on something else. Each study had a specific purpose, they made their conclusions, and then moved on to another study. Nobody was taking this little gem from one study and what was learned from another study, saying, "What if we tried this, combined with that?" Jay spent the next eight years doing exactly that, and now as a result, we have very special, one-of-a-kind wearable neurotechnology that changes lives every single day.

You simply wear the socks or put the insoles in your shoes, and the moment that happens, our technology begins to impact your brain. You will have improved balance, more strength, and greater range of motion.

I know, you're probably saying, "Yeah, right." But one of the greatest things about this technology is that it begins to happen instantly. It's drug-free, non-invasive, and perhaps best of all, affordable and guaranteed. We put our money where your feet are. Everyone is welcome to try it themselves and if for any reason you're not completely satisfied, you get a refund. And I can tell you, in our two and a half years on the market, our return rate is less than one percent. It's the opposite that happens; people call and say, "I need more. I want some for my mom, my aunt, my kids, and my neighbor with Parkinson's." It has been very rewarding.

My phone rings every day with people just calling to say, "Thank you for telling me about these socks. You're not going to believe what just happened to my mom." I have spent the past two years traveling the country showing this product, tipping people over, and letting them experience it for themselves. The stories never end. I can't make up stories as good as the real-life experiences I see and hear about our socks. I've been to over 20 medical conferences ranging from physical therapy, to chiropractic, to neurological, to optometric—you name it. I've given each of these doctors and practitioners the same four-word pitch: "Take off your shoes," just like I did with my mom. I have even been in the boardroom with Dr. Oz and asked him to take off his shoes and tipped him over. He stepped on the insoles, and I could not budge him. I've done this over 12,000 times and it happens each time. It's as if I can see the wheels turning in their head as they think of everyone they want to share this with.

This story has become very personal for me. A year ago, my mom was in a beautiful assisted living facility. She had just woken up, was getting out of bed, slipped, and fell. They rushed her to the ER and determined that she broke her hip. While she was not a great candidate for surgery, the surgeon told us that without it, she will never even be able to sit up in bed. She wanted to try, so they operated. The hip replacement was a success, but she never fully recovered from the anesthesia, and eight days later she was gone.

You hear stories like this all the time. According to government statistics, if someone 70 or older breaks a hip, over 50 percent of that population will not make it past 12 months. I understand how falling is a critical problem for our geriatric population, and I want to do everything I can to help share this amazing technology to help reduce their risk of falling and improve their quality of life.

If you're lucky enough to still have parents or elders in your life, give them some of our socks; it's the ultimate gift. Watch the expression on their face when you try to gently tip them over, or you see an improvement in their gait and mobility. It's a life changer! Check out our website. We actually have over 40,000 testimonials. We have curated a handful of videos that begin to tell the story, but you can dive deeper and watch as many as you want. You'll see tremors reduced, improved balance, people on walkers, stroke survivors, improved range of motion, and instant, remarkable outcomes in thousands of other real-life people.

We feel our product has benefits for everyone, not just those with balance issues. Name one sport that wouldn't benefit from an improvement in balance, strength, and range of motion. Golfers, batters, and hockey players love this product. In fact, on my website you will see videos from the LA Kings, the USC athletic department, three-time world champion men's figure skater, Elvis Stojko, a young PGA golfer, and more.

Because what we're doing is neurological and not mechanical, some of the impacts are dramatic. Do you happen to know anyone with kids on the autism spectrum? If so, give them some socks! We have hundreds of stories from parents and grandparents who tell us, "The moment little Johnny puts on his socks, it's as if there's a calming effect that comes over him." We hear similar outcomes with ADHD and adults with PTSD.

We should note that our socks and insoles don't treat, diagnose, or cure any disease. Nothing we do or say should be considered a substitute for consultation, examination, and treatment by your healthcare professional.

So, what's the secret to our products? We call it Voxx HPT, "Human Performance Technology."

It's a proprietary pattern of neuro-stimulation. Some people think of it as "reflexology to go." For thousands of years, Chinese medicine has known the significance of the bottom of the feet. The soles of your feet are filled with neuroreceptors that aid the brain in proprioception. This is the brain's ability to basically defy gravity and keep us upright. Picture yourself standing barefoot on a white, sandy beach in Hawaii. There is a constant pathway of millions of impulses from special nerves in your muscles and joints that provide information to your brain about tension, position, and location. Information from your big toe, your little toe, and your knee is being sent to and from the brain, which has to constantly figure out where to add pressure, where to relax a muscle, and how much to contract a joint. Whether you're trying to simply stand up, walk, run, bend over, or balance on one foot, it's a nonstop task for the brain to make it happen. Many things can complicate this journey. Whether it's injury, age, or disease, there are thousands of issues that can have a detrimental impact on your balance.

By wearing our socks or insoles, our special pattern helps provide more sensory input to the brain, helping to edge it towards homeostasis. Think of a garage door opener. If you're in your driveway and you press the button, the door opens. But if you're in a neighbor's driveway and press the button on your opener, their door doesn't open because you don't have the right code. Jay cracked the code for every human on the planet. The same pattern will stimulate the neuropathway for everyone, another reason why this is such a remarkable product.

When you look at the bottom of our socks, you'll see what looks like an orange fingerprint. It is actually Jay's fingerprint, which is an interesting story. Our attorneys said there were two ways to protect our intellectual property. We could file patents, but in today's day and age, you publish your patents and then you have to be prepared for people trying to rip you off and you spend lots of time and money trying to defend your patents and getting people to cease and desist from infringement. The other option is to keep your technology a secret, like the formula for Coca-Cola or the recipe for Kentucky Fried Chicken. We all know there's 11 secret herbs and spices, but we don't know exactly which ones and in what amounts. Thus, we hid our special pattern within Jay's fingerprint and filed international copyrights. If anyone tries to steal it, it's not only an international copyright violation, but it also constitutes identity theft—a very clever legal strategy.

How our technology works is not as important as that it works. That being said, we love skeptics. We invite you to read some of the studies, look at the brain scans, and dig as deep as you want into the research and theory. It is too complex to explain here, we still have neurologists scratching their heads. As they will tell you, the brain is the biggest mystery in the Universe, and medical science learns new things about the brain every day.

But as they say, the best proof is seeing it with your own eyes and feeling it with your own feet. While studies are great and the "gold standard" is a randomized, placebo-controlled, double-blind study is a great way to help determine and demonstrate efficacy of a drug or treatment protocol, there is also the old adage that it didn't take a double-blind, placebo-controlled study to figure out that wearing a parachute really works. You don't need to have a hundred people jump from a plane without a parachute and compare the end result with the 100 people who jumped with a parachute.

Please order some of our socks and insoles and try it. Be a mensch and order some for the people in your life and watch what happens. They will thank you. Do your own investigation; it's quick and profound. You can help us improve lives. Who would have thought that something as simple as changing your socks could change your life?

I sincerely thank you and hope to hear some of the amazing stories of what happens to the people in your life. Together we can improve the quality of life for millions (okay, billions) of people.

Thank you.

About the Author

Stan Esecson

Stan has spent his career helping others achieve their goals. With over 40 years of marketing expertise, he has worked with a wide range of clients ranging from the most famous wineries in the world, top hotels, and start-up entrepreneurs.

Contact Information:
Telephone: (949) 547-1683
Websites: www.SeeOurSocksinAction.com
            www.SeeOurSocksinAction.net

About the Editor

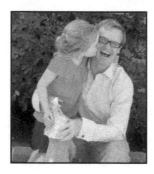

Steven E. Schmitt

Steven E has made over 1,000 books bestsellers. He can make your book a bestseller on BarnesandNoble.com, Amazon.com or even on the *New York Times* book list.

He has worked with world-renowned authors, top doctors, CEOs of major companies, top fiction and non-fiction authors, and owners of top franchises. He loves helping authors, who have a powerful message, learn how to get it out to the world.

Go to www.bestsellerguru.com for your FREE book, *How I Sold Millions of Books.*

You can find more information go to my YouTube channel:
bestsellerguru
[over 100 book marketing videos]

email Steven at:
Selawofpositivity@gmail.com

or call Steven on:
1-562-884-0062
(I will do my best to get back to you as soon as I can but remember I'm very busy with authors from around the world)